MULTIPLE SCLEROSIS

FORTHCOMING TITLES

Occupational Therapy for the Brain-Injured Adult
Jo Clark-Wilson and Gordon Muir Giles

Modern Electrotherapy
Mary Dyson and Christopher Hayne

Autism
A multidisciplinary approach
Edited by Kathryn Ellis

Limb Amputation
From aetiology to rehabilitation
Rosalind Ham and Leonard Cotton

Physiotherapy in Respiratory and Intensive Care
Alexandra Hough

Understanding Dysphasia
Lesley Jordan and Rita Twiston Davies

Management in Occupational Therapy
Zielfa B. Maslin

Dysarthria
Theory and therapy
Sandra J. Robertson

Occupational Therapy in Rheumatology
Lynne Sandlers

Speech and Language Problems in Children
Dilys A. Treharne

THERAPY IN PRACTICE SERIES

Edited by Jo Campling

This series of books is aimed at 'therapists' concerned with rehabilitation in a very broad sense. The intended audience particularly includes occupational therapists, physiotherapists and speech therapists, but many titles will also be of interest to nurses, psychologists, medical staff, social workers, teachers or volunteer workers. Some volumes are interdisciplinary, others are aimed at one particular profession. All titles will be comprehensive but concise, and practical but with due reference to relevant theory and evidence. They are not research monographs but focus on professional practice, and will be of value to both students and qualified personnel.

Multiple Sclerosis
Approaches to Management

LORRAINE DE SOUZA
Research Co-ordinator, ARMS Unit
Central Middlesex Hospital

In association with
Action and Research for Multiple Sclerosis

CHAPMAN AND HALL

LONDON • NEW YORK • TOKYO • MELBOURNE • MADRAS

UK	Chapman and Hall, 2–6 Boundary Row, London SE1 8HN
USA	Chapman and Hall, 29 West 35th Street, New York NY10001
JAPAN	Chapman and Hall Japan, Thomson Publishing Japan, Hirakawacho Nemoto Building, 7F, 1-7-11 Hirakawa-cho, Chiyoda-ku, Tokyo 102
AUSTRALIA	Chapman and Hall Australia, Thomas Nelson Australia, 480 La Trobe Street, PO Box 4725, Melbourne 3000
INDIA	Chapman and Hall India, R. Seshadri, 32 Second Main Road, CIT East, Madras 600 035

First edition 1990

© 1990 Lorraine De Souza

Typeset in 10/12pt Times by Mayhew Typesetting, Bristol
Printed in Great Britain by St Edmundsbury Press Ltd,
Bury St Edmunds, Suffolk

ISBN 0 412 32230 7

British Library Cataloguing in Publication Data

De Souza, Lorraine
  Multiple sclerosis.
  1. Man. Multiple sclerosis. Therapy
  I. Title II. Action and Research for Multiple Sclerosis
  III. Series
  616.83406

  ISBN 0–412–32230–7

Library of Congress Cataloging-in-Publication Data

Multiple sclerosis: approaches to management / [edited by]
  Lorraine De Souza in association with Action and Research for
  Multiple Sclerosis. – 1st ed.
    p. cm. – (Therapy in practice series: 18)
  Includes bibliographical references.
  ISBN 0–412–32230–7
  1. Multiple sclerosis. 2. Multiple sclerosis – Physical therapy.
3. Occupational therapy. I. De Souza, Lorraine, 1955– .
II. Action and Research for Multiple Sclerosis. III. Series.
  [DNLM: 1. Multiple Sclerosis – therapy. WL 360 M95637]
RC377.M844 1990
616.8′3406–dc20
DNLM/DLC   90-1790
for Library of Congress   CIP

Dedicated to the members
of Action and Research for
Multiple Sclerosis (ARMS)

Contents

Contributors

Lorraine H. De Souza, MSc, MCSP Grad, Dip, Phys.
Research Co-ordinator and Superintendent Physiotherapist
(Research)
ARMS Research Unit, Central Middlesex Hospital

Pam Enderby, PhD, LCST
Chief Speech Therapist,
Frenchay Hospital, Bristol

Geraldine Fitzgerald, BSc. PhD.
Former Research Nutritionist,
ARMS Research Unit, Central Middlesex Hospital

Rosemary Jones, BSc, Ph.D.
Research Fellow, Biophysics Group,
Radiotherapy and Oncology Centre, Bristol Royal Infirmary

Leo Lange, MD, FRCP
Consultant Neurologist
Formerly at Charing Cross Hospital, London

Judith Monks, MA, B. Nurs.
Research Fellow,
Brunel ARMS Unit, Department of Human Sciences, Brunel
University

Ian Robinson, MA
Director,
Brunel ARMS Unit, Department of Human Sciences, Brunel
University

Julia Segal, MA
Research Counsellor,
ARMS Research Unit, Central Middlesex Hospital

Kay Smithers, BN, RGN, RHV
Former Lecturer,
Department Nursing Studies, University of Wales College of
Medicine, Cardiff

Jennifer Worthington, MPT, MCSP
Superintendent Research Physiotherapist,
ARMS Research Unit, Central Middlesex Hospital

Acknowledgements

Thanks go to all the contributing authors, especially those who have contributed original work. Special thanks go to Ann Ashburn, who has allowed me to use work we have done together, both published and unpublished. Avril Plunkett, MBAOT, has provided valuable discussion and advice for the chapter on Occupational Therapy for which I am grateful, and Judith Monks has helped with the concluding chapter. Particular help is acknowledged from my colleague Jennifer Worthington for many useful discussions and suggestions, and from Action and Research for Multiple Sclerosis (ARMS) which has supported much of the work described in the book. Finally, my thanks go to Margaret Blindell and Jocelyn Warner for typing and word processing.

The royalties from this publication will be donated to the Charity, Action and Research for Multiple Sclerosis, and the contributing authors are thanked for their generosity.

Lorraine H. De Souza
ARMS Research Unit
Central Middlesex Hospital
London NW10

January 1990

1

Managing multiple sclerosis: A partnership between professional practitioners and patients

Ian Robinson

Multiple sclerosis as a disease is a medical puzzle. Its aetiology is unknown, it is problematic to diagnose at an early stage, difficult to offer sound and accurate prognoses for individuals, and there is no cure. If affects more women than men, usually with onset in early adulthood, and is distinguished epidemiologically by a distinct geographical distribution with a concentration of cases in the temperate latitudes of the world (Acheson, 1985). As a very broad generalization, it appears that the prevalence rate is approximately six in 10 000 people in these temperate latitudes – Europe, N. America, Japan and Australasia (Gonzalez-Scarano, Spielman and Nathanson, 1986) – although there are smaller areas of far higher prevalence (Kurtzke and Hyllested, 1979; Poskanzer *et al.,* 1980). Sensory and functional systems are affected in varying degrees over an unpredictable course in a condition which is often characterized by relapses and remissions (Matthews, 1985a). Other cases show a slow progression over many years (Compston, 1987). In these cases a normal life span is not substantially jeopardized, although increasingly severe disability may occur. In a small number of cases a more rapid course is evident, leading to death more quickly after onset (Carter, Sciarra and Merritt, 1950).

From this brief description it can be seen that managing multiple sclerosis (MS) is a complex task for all those involved with the disease. This complexity arises from a wide range of factors which, in their variety and nature, are unique to the condition, and its clinical, social and individual consequences.

The clinical symptoms and signs evident in the disease may variably affect almost all body functions at different times in different ways. As Matthews (1985b) notes:

> The diversity of symptoms, signs and course of multiple sclerosis . . . continues to astonish even the most experienced physician . . . (p.146)

In addition, in the absence of a clear aetiology, and a cure for the condition, the professional practitioner is faced with understanding its particular physical effects, differentiating those from the effects of other unrelated conditions, and providing symptomatic management in as ameliorative a way as possible (see Chapter 2).

However, there are further complexities in this process of managing MS. Clinically observed signs and symptoms as manifestations of an organic pathology in the course of the disease may only prove to be a partial guide to the functional consequences for individuals. Therefore it is not always clear, particularly in the early stages of the disease, to what extent observed functional problems are directly the result of neurological damage. In the later stages of the condition, functional consequences are not necessarily uniform for all individuals even with what appear to be similar and severe levels of impairment (Matthews, 1985b).

Even when the functional consequences of MS can be readily traced to a distinctly neurological origin, the social and individual meaning of the consequences for those affected may be quite different (see Chapter 10). Patients may have very different priorities and life goals. Thus the same functional problems may result in dissimilar effects on each of their lives. For example, although loss of mobility, deterioration in sight, or an inability to write, present problems for all those affected, the individual and personal consequences for each patient may be significantly different (Robinson, 1988a). In short, it is problematic to assume that a known physical lesion with particular functional consequences will be interpreted and prioritized in the same way by each patient. On a related point, a patient's own priorities may well be different from those of clinicians and other professional staff (Baer and Lewis, 1987). In addition, patients live in a social world where they have families, partners or others with whom they share their lives. Such people will have their own ideas about the problems arising from the disease and what should be achieved in managing the condition, both for the person with MS, and for themselves (Lincoln, 1981). Discrepancies in interpretations and priorities, and thus conflicts, can easily be generated in this situation between those with the disease, family members and professional staff, in establishing how, and by whom, the disease should be managed.

Therefore, in a clinical setting, the intrusion of personal and social factors may not only be difficult to avoid, but such factors may substantially influence the outcome of professional strategies. In a range of conditions it has been demonstrated that the successful redress of particular functional problems will be influenced by the personal motivation and social situation of the patient (Green, Pratt and Grigsby, 1984; Thompson and Haran, 1984; Tyerman and Humphrey, 1984). Moreover, some patients will still continue to experience major problems of personal adjustment even following the relatively beneficial outcome of functional management (Field, Cordle and Bowman, 1983). Therefore there is, perhaps disappointingly, no automatic and positive relationship between a resolution or improvement in functional status and the broader quality of life of a patient or their family. It appears that there can be a greater independence between the successful management of functional problems of a physical kind, and individual and social well-being, than had been previously thought.

The managerial task in relation to MS is therefore not an easy one to define, or to categorize rigidly. In addition to this general interlocking of personal, social and functional problems, their multifaceted and changing nature will draw on the skills of many different disciplines in different phases of the disease process. Thus the coordination of those interventions and their smooth organization is of concern. As each of the therapeutic interventions may deal with some special aspect of physical or psychological disorder, the ways in which they are linked and the transition between them is particularly important. The common denominator in this process is the patient and there is a persuasive case for encouraging a more systematic incorporation of the patient's perspective in the continuing and difficult task of successfully managing MS.

THE IDEA OF PARTNERSHIP IN THE MANAGEMENT OF MS

It has always been a particular irritation for therapists and others professionally concerned with the management of conditions like MS that therapies which appear in professional terms to be for the patient's own good may not be adopted at all by patients, or are employed by them only sporadically or partially.

Research suggests that much formal medical advice in relation to all sorts of conditions, let alone in relation to advice from therapists, is not followed by patients (Thompson, 1984a). Appointments may be missed (Sackett and Snow, 1979), recommendations may be ignored (Thompson, 1984a; pp. 113–14), prescribed medicines may not be taken (Feinstein *et al.,* 1959), other actions considered appropriate may not be pursued, especially those requiring patients' cooperation outside immediate and direct medical control (Ley, 1977, 1978).

The general problem denoted by this issue – that is, the difference between professionally recommended therapeutic actions and what patients actually do – is that which is usually called the problem of compliance. There is a burgeoning literature on this issue (Ley, 1988) which both documents the extent of non-compliance, and indicates strategies which may minimize it. However, strategies for reducing non-compliance which may be appropriate in acute and medically remediable conditions, and where patients are under direct medical supervision, are generally less effective in long-term chronic conditions like MS where patients have to pursue most of the management of the condition outside continuous medical control.

This suggests that an understanding and appreciation of patients' own goals and objectives in their management of MS is a necessary component of successful professional management of the disease. In this context it is important to consider the ways in which both therapists and patients acquire their knowledge about how to manage conditions like MS.

Formal training and education in the technical skills of patient management and care is typical of all the professions associated with chronic diseases like MS. Through such processes, relevant procedures and their contingent effects are learnt and practised. In theory, the techniques used are those that have withstood the test of scientific examination and have emerged as the most profitable in remedying functional or other problems. In practice, scientifically proven techniques are interwoven with those which on less formal practical criteria are deemed to be helpful to the management of patients. However, it is not only professional staff who are trained in managing problems of illness.

It must be recognized that patients and their families have also learnt how to deal with illness in their lives, through the training provided by family and friends, and through trial and error from their own experiences (Locker, 1981). Each person has developed a series of strategies by which they deal with their own health problems (Calnan, 1987). Some of these may be general to most people in a society, others may be particular and individual. These strategies condition how and in what circumstances people with health problems seek professional help (Cornwell, 1984). Studies have shown how most health care does not involve professional advice or support, and even people with medically serious conditions may not seek medical advice because their priorities and perceptions are at variance with those of the formal health care system (McEwan, Martini and Wilkins, 1983; Chapter 5). It is understandable therefore in relation to MS that it may take some time for people with mild and early symptoms to enter the medical system, as they may initially deal with the symptoms themselves or they may perceive them at first as unrelated to serious illness (Stewart and Sullivan, 1982). The factors which precipitate the seeking of medical support will thus vary considerably between individuals, as well as being reciprocally dependent on the perceived efficacy of the formal health services (Robinson, 1988b).

Given the absence of any clear therapy which can be medically recommended which will cure MS, it is perhaps unsurprising that people subsequently diagnosed as having the condition will have their own ideas about how it should be managed. Such ideas may be drawn from the previous ways in which they have managed their own 'MS-like' symptoms, or be more generally drawn from a range of extra-medical sources which seem to them to have a practical relevance to their situation (Robinson, 1988b). Such ideas may arise from, or be recommended by family members, friends, other people with MS, self-help organizations and the media. These ideas can, and do, differ from those frequently considered medically appropriate. The personal ideas and practices are just as likely to be part of a patient's continuing individual life style, as they are to be the result of any general antipathy to medicine or medical practice.

Therapists and doctors may be concerned about, and perhaps dismissive of, the unconventional therapies or strategies used by patients in managing MS, and thus will ignore them and the reasons why they are adopted (Davis, 1966). However, there is little evidence that these attitudes either result in a substantial reduction of those therapies deemed professionally inappropriate, or result over time in an increase in the use of professionally recommended therapies. Professional assertions of benefit may increase a patient's compliance in the short term, but the overall relationship between medical authority and compliance is complex (Thompson, 1984a). A more profitable approach to what is likely to be a long-term condition, is to seek to understand the basis on which both medically recommended and unconventional therapies are used by patients. Through such an approach the emphasis is shifted from non-compliance being a result of a patient's problematic personal qualities, to non-compliance being the result of difficulties in the relationship between therapist and patient for which each party bears some responsibility (Stone, 1979).

To consider this issue in a different way, the consultations between therapists and patients may be described as 'Meetings between Experts' (Tuckett *et al.*, 1985) in which the professional expertise of therapists is complemented by the experience of patients in their knowledge of their own condition, and how their lives are affected by it. The partnership implied here indicates that patients acknowledge the specific professional skills of therapists, while therapists recognize the unique position of patients to use and interpret those skills in the light of their own life goals. Fundamentally, a partnership would recognize the individual circumstances of patients not only in terms of their differing functional problems, but also in terms of their attitudes, feelings and objectives about the relative importance of possibly competing strategies. Such an approach may be innovative for some therapists whose training and focus has traditionally been based on their skills in ameliorating particular functional problems. It may also be innovative for some patients who have been shown to be reluctant to communicate information about aspects of their symptoms and their coping strategies, which may be important for effective professional intervention (Thompson, 1984b). However, it may be the only approach which ensures that patients continue to pursue a mutually agreed set of strategies when they are outside the immediate control of the therapist.

THE MANAGEMENT OF MS BY THE THERAPIST AND THE PATIENT: WHOSE RESPONSIBILITY IS IT?

The idea of partnership not only suggests an acknowledgement of the different goals that patients and therapists may have in relation to MS, but also that the responsibility for the management of the condition will be shared as well. Such ideas raise a range of important possibilities, as well as a range of practical difficulties.

From the comments made earlier it seems clear that many people with MS have already 'taken responsibility' for their condition, by making their own decisions as to when and in what circumstances they entered into the medical system in the first place. Further, such people are likely to continue to be actively involved in seeking and personally assessing therapies, and acceding to them after learning their diagnosis (Cunningham, 1977).

However, some patients may have a different managerial approach which minimizes the salience of the disease in their lives (commonly perceived as denial – Matson and Brooks, 1977) making the

6

intervention of therapists particularly problematic. Yet others may appear to surrender personal control of the disease to the authority of the doctor and therapist, creating equal difficulties in its effective management. In this latter situation the patient may firmly place responsibility for the successful outcome of therapy, as well as blame for its failure, on those professionally involved. Such an attitude may be counter-productive for treatments requiring active participation, especially outside a hospital and within a community setting.

In theory, in the absence of a cure for the disease, persons with MS should be able to draw on professional assistance and advice as required, to aid them to live with their condition and its symptomatic manifestations. Similarly, the family of such a person should be able to obtain professional assistance to manage their own day-to-day difficulties. Within this model the responsibility for the management of the condition is firstly that of the patient, and only when this personal management is undermined or breaks down does it devolve either on other family members or professional help.

In practice the situation is far more complicated. Individuals with MS often want to take responsibility for their lives and the treatments they pursue. At other times they may want someone else to take responsibility. Members of the family may 'take over', or may fail to take what others think to be reasonable responsibility. Similarly, different professionals involved with the management of MS – consultants, general practitioners, physiotherapists, district nurses, occupational therapists and others – may each at times wish to take responsibility, but at other times devolve that responsibility to others. What each 'manager' does may influence how other professional support is given. The way that responsibility is allocated and changed may, given the health service and professional boundaries, have relatively little to do with the precise nature of the presenting problems, and perhaps may have even less to do with the wishes of patients, or their families (Elian and Dean, 1983).

At critical points there may be differences of opinion as to who has the responsibility, or the competence, to undertake critical managerial tasks. Communicating the diagnosis, for example, although frequently seen as the consultant's prerogative, may in effect be delegated to others, as may the giving of crucial information to patients and their families about life choices – such as whether to have children (Elian and Dean, 1985). One of the problems in this kind of setting, and with this kind of information giving, is that only rarely can categorical advice be given. Often information is of a probabilistic and uncertain kind, as indeed may be the case when attempting to predict the effects of therapies in individual cases. Thus there may be 'rational' disagreements over whether one course of action should be taken rather than another, as well as conflicts over 'irrational' sets of values, beliefs and behaviours which, for patients and their families, may make one kind of outcome far more desirable than others.

The question of responsibility for the management of MS also has another dimension. For the most part, professional expertise and thus responsibility is confined within recognized limits; indeed the maintenance of a clear professional identity is largely dependent on gaining an effective monopoly over a body of knowledge and practice. However, even in relation to an apparently discreet and bounded professional role, many factors intervene which make such boundaries difficult to live within. Within professions such as physiotherapy or occupational therapy there may be quite different views about the relationship with the patient or client. For some the professional role focuses on the effective application of a technique to a particular set of functional problems, for example, defective muscular movements which, if cumulatively remedied, would lead to a better capacity to perform certain everyday tasks (Alaszewski, 1979). For others the professional role focuses on the overall quality of life of the whole person, in which case technical skills may be applied quite differently (Hall, 1987).

Each working model of the professional relationship presupposes to a large degree that the outcome of the therapy depends on the motivation of the patient, as well as on the approach and skills of the therapist. The approach of the therapist, and indeed the usual criteria by which success is measured, may need considerable re-evaluation in the case of MS. In relation to such a progressive disease therapeutic interventions take place against the background of possible continuing functional loss for many patients, even though there is increasing evidence that some dietary and other therapies may have a role in stabilizing certain aspects of the condition (see Chapter 8). However, the variability of the course of MS is such as to confound an easy and singular approach to intervention. For some therapists this may be a professionally difficult situation to manage, or a situation which is deemed less prestigious than the management of some acute conditions in which dramatic amelioration of functional deficits may be possible.

The complex way in which managing a chronic condition like MS must be undertaken raises further questions about the nature of the professional role. The presence at any one time of a series of inter-linked problems – functional, social or personal – may transcend any particular professional boundary. To what extent is there a duty to identify and seek to solve problems, even if such problems are outside a particular sphere of professional expertise? Where do individual professional roles begin and end? Is it helpful to identify issues for which there is little professional help available? The variable distribution of professional resources, different visions of professional responsibilities, difficulties over the coordination of services and inadequate communication between individuals may lead to relatively arbitrary resolution of these questions.

There may also be additional costs in terms of professional time and resources involved in extending the focus of responsibility for those concerned with people with MS. Many underlying personal or emotional problems of patients may lead to the extension of the professional role apparently beyond the therapist's ordinary expecta-tions. Thus the extent to which any individual therapist or doctor can probe into all the possible problems linked with MS may be limited, and their revelation and solution may in the end be left to the patient or the patient's family. Yet the uncovering of these problems, and their management, could be vital for the comfortable continuation of the therapist/patient relationship, and for the resolution of how physical or functional difficulties can best be met.

Finally, it is important to reiterate that the uncertainties endemic in the management of the disease considerably complicate the task of taking professional responsibility. In the unpredictable development of the condition the therapist, as well as the patient and the patient's family, may feel a frustrating lack of control over the effects of their actions.

UNDERSTANDING THE PATIENT IN MANAGING MS

Some points of difference and possible points of conflict between therapists and patients and their families in the management of MS have already been identified. At one level everyone is dealing with the same problem – the disease. At another level, as has already been noted, the meaning and effects of the condition can be substan-tially different.

The question of what causes MS and hence how it may be con-trolled is of interest to different people in different ways. The classification and ordering of diseases, their associated symptoms and signs, and their possible causes is an intrinsic part of medical endeavour. For professional purposes the classificatory process is in many respects both an end in itself – as a necessary mechanism for identifying each disease with precision – as well as an immediate means to other ends, such as developing better treatments. In the longer term any acquisition of scientific knowledge about MS, however esoteric from the point of view of everyday management of the condition, is a positive virtue in developing possible future therapies. However, the current discrepancy between the accretion of broad scientific information about the disease and the relative inadequacy of present methods of control presents special difficulties for both patients and therapists. For professional staff faced with the pressure of accommodating the hopes and fears of patients, there are difficulties over admitting the incompleteness of present knowledge, over the problem of the relatively poor prediction of individual outcomes, over the inadequacy of managerial strategies in the light of hopes for a cure, and perhaps also over personal feelings of professional inadequacy in this setting. Thus there may be a temptation to overplay the certainties in interactions with patients, to cover over, at least initially, the longer-term problems. However, the day-to-day management exercised by patients and their families over the condition needs as accurate information for its effective use as does medical science for effective research. Although well-intentioned overstated indications of professional certainty may prove only a temporary palliative, such an approach may eventually rebound on the same or other staff.

However, there may be certain circumstances in which the onus for managing the condition is placed firmly on the therapist by the patient. Here there is an expectation of authoritative advice, whether or not such advice can legitimately be given. In such cases the patient hands over the control of the condition to the therapist. It may be even more important in such a situation to resist the challenge to take on complete responsibility for a situation which cannot effectively be professionally remedied without the active participation of the patient.

One of the major differences between the approach of patients, their families and professionals to managing MS is the personal focus of the patient to that management. At a general level people may be interested in broad information about MS, such as how many people it affects, where they live and how old they are. However, running through this concern is a more particular focus on themselves and their own situation. There is therefore in this process a translation of the global into the individual, and a transformation of the general into the personal. For therapists and others this can be a difficult issue to deal with. Questions of prognosis, for example, which are problematic even in general terms, may only be meaningful to individuals insofar as their own chances of deterioration are specifically indicated. Questions of the general effects of therapeutic intervention – through physiotherapy or speech therapy for example – will be interpreted in terms of the likelihood of specific personal effects by the patient or client. This personalizing of expectations and contacts compared with those professionally concerned with managing MS is understandable. After all, in the patient's eyes, it is not MS in the abstract that is being managed, but MS as embodied in themselves and their lives which is the focus of their attention.

This point raises another issue, which is the particular way in which information is likely to be communicated by patients to therapists and doctors about their condition. The nature of the symptoms occurring in MS is such that they are often difficult for some patients to describe in terms which are clearly identifiable to therapists and doctors – especially those which involve sensory problems. On the other hand many of those with a chronic condition acquire detailed medical terminology for their symptoms in the course of their contact with the medical system. Indeed, on occasion patients may possess more medical and scientific information about MS than some of the professional staff with whom they come into contact. Such knowledge in itself can be very forbidding, perhaps even threatening to a therapist or a general practitioner whose acquaintance with patients with the disease has been occasional rather than sustained.

One additional feature associated with people with MS which may also create potential difficulties in relation to professional intervention, is the unusually vigorous role that they may take in managing their condition, over and above that associated with other progressive diseases (Pollack, 1984). People with MS often refer to 'fighting the disease' (Cunningham, 1977), and through their purposive and, for others, perhaps aggressive search for a therapy which may help them, may not afford any privileged status to professionally endorsed therapies. This factor, combined with the often sophisticated knowledge of the condition mentioned above, may make negotiations over the exact role of professional therapies problematic, especially from a therapist's point of view. However, such an active search for therapies may not necessarily be endorsed by other family members of the patient whose view of the patient's functional problems, and their managerial strategies, may be very different (Robinson, 1988c). Individual family members may have their own everyday goals in relation to which, for example, involvement in strenuous attempts to maintain a patient's very marginal capacity for mobility is viewed very negatively. Thus the rehabilitative objectives of patients and their families may not be as congruent as Power (1985) suggests. For a therapist it may not be possible therefore to count on the active support of family members for any treatment that is recommended in the interests of the patient. This indicates that in establishing the most effective conditions for successful therapy, positive negotiations with key family members may be just as important as negotiations with the patient.

THE THERAPIST AND THE PATIENT IN THE MANAGEMENT OF MS

One of the most important features of almost all therapies for symptoms of MS is that they require the active cooperation of patients to be successful. Whilst particular emphasis has been placed on the importance of the therapist understanding the patient's personal and social situation to ensure the best chances of successful treatment, it is equally important for patients to realistically appraise the contribution that therapists can make to the management of their condition.

However understanding and perceptive therapists may be, it can be difficult for some patients to benefit from their skills. Patients may overestimate the extent to which therapists can control or ameliorate their problems; they may focus their own concern or anger over the disease or its consequences on the relationship with the therapist; they may not perceive the importance of their own day-to-day behaviour in reinforcing the recommendations of therapists; they may not understand that a professional intervention is often of limited duration for specific purposes, and not for an unlimited time and for a range of purposes; they may transform the relationship from one centred around functional problems to one centred almost entirely around personal or emotional problems; or they may refuse to acknowledge key aspects of their disease, which is a necessary precondition for effective therapy.

In such circumstances, where misunderstandings and difficulties may quickly arise from misconceptions at the start of the relationship between therapists and their patients with MS, it is important to negotiate in advance the basis on which the relationship will proceed. Establishing a contract after an initial assessment, if necessary in writing, and specifying the obligations of each of the parties to the therapeutic relationship, is one way of minimizing initial discrepancies in expectations. By indicating such factors as the number and timing of the consultations, the specific and agreed objective(s) of the relationship, the obligations of the patient (and the family) to continue appropriate activities between sessions, and the length of the contract, allows many potential problems between therapist and patient to be identified and in many cases resolved. This contract can be re-negotiated or renewed with the agreement of all those concerned. In such a contract the partnership between therapist and patient is clearly enshrined in an agreement which allows less room for initial misunderstandings and problems. If flexibly employed it may enable therapy in a complex condition like MS to be far more effectively undertaken, by placing the onus jointly on the patient and the therapist, thus producing a genuine partnership.

REFERENCES

Acheson, E.D. (1985) The pattern of the disease, in *McAlpine's Multiple Sclerosis*. W.B. Matthews, E.D. Acheson, J.R. Batchelor and R.O. Weller. Churchill Livingstone, London, pp. 3–26.

Alaszewski, A.E. (1979) Rehabilitation, the remedial therapy professions and social policy. *Social Science and Medicine* **13**, 431–43.

Baer, G. and Lewis, Y. (1987) The rehabilitation of a severely disabled multiple sclerosis patient. *Physiotherapy*, **73**, 436–8.

Calnan, M. (1987) *Health and Illness: The lay perspective*. Tavistock, London.

Carter, S., Sciarra, D. and Merritt, H.H. (1950) The course of multiple sclerosis determined by autopsy proven cases. *Research Publications of the Association for Research into Nervous and Mental Diseases,* **28**, 471–511.

Compston, A. (1987) Can the course of multiple sclerosis be predicted? in *More Dilemmas in Neurology* (eds C.P. Warian and J.S. Garfield). Churchill Livingstone, Edinburgh.

Cornwell, J. (1984) *Hard Earned Lives: Accounts of health and illness from East London*. Tavistock. London.

Cunningham, D.J. (1977) Stigma and social isolation: self-perceived problems of a group of multiple sclerosis sufferers. Rep.27, Health Services Research Unit, Centre for Research in the Social Sciences, University of Kent.

Davis, M.S. (1966) Variations in patients' compliance with doctors' orders: analysis of congruence between survey responses and the results of empirical investigations. *Journal of Medical Education,* **41**, 1037–48.

Elian, M. and Dean, G. (1983) Need for and use of social and health services by multiple sclerosis patients in England and Wales. *Lancet* i, (No.8333) 14 May, 1091–3.

Elian, M. and Dean, G. (1985) To tell or not to tell the diagnosis of multiple sclerosis. *Lancet* ii, 6 July, 27–8.

Feinstein, A.R., Wood, H.F., Epstein, J.A. *et al.* (1959) A controlled study of three methods of prophylaxis against streptococcal infection in a population of rheumatic children. II. Results of the first three years of the study. *New England Journal of Medicine,* **260**, 697–702.

Field, D., Cordle, C.J. and Bowman, G.S. (1983) Coping with stroke at home. *International Rehabilitation Medicine,* **5**, 96–100.

Gonzalez-Scarano, F., Spielman, R.S. and Nathanson, N. (1986) Epidemiology, in *Multiple Sclerosis* (eds W.I. McDonald and D.H. Silberberg). Butterworths, London, pp. 37–55.

Green, B.C., Pratt, C.C. and Grigsby, T.E. (1984) Self concept amongst persons with long-term spinal cord injury. *Archives of Physical Medicine and Rehabilitation,* **65**, 751–4.

Hall, M. (1987) Models of occupational therapy. M.Phil. thesis, Brunel University.

Kurtzke, J.F. and Hyllested, K. (1979) Multiple sclerosis in the Faroe Islands. 1. Clinical and epidemiological features. *Annals of Neurology,* **5**, 6–21.

Ley, P. (1977) Towards better doctor–patient communication: contributions from social and experimental psychology, in *Communications Between Doctors and Patients* (ed. A.E. Bennett) Nuffield Provincial Hospitals Trust, London.

Ley, P. (1978) Psychological and behavioural factors in weight loss, in *Recent Advances in Obesity Research* (ed. G.A. Bray) Vol.2. Newman Publishing, London.

Ley, P. (1988) Communication between doctors and patients. Chapman and Hall, London.

Lincoln, N.B. (1981) Discrepancies between capabilities and performance of activities of daily living in multiple sclerosis patients. *International Rehabilitation Medicine,* **3**, 84–8.

Locker, D. (1981) *Symptoms and Illness.* Tavistock, London.

McEwan, J., Martini, C.J.M. and Wilkins, N. (1983) *Participation in Health.* Croom Helm, London.

Matson, R.R. and Brooks, N.A. (1977) Adjusting to multiple sclerosis: An exploratory study. *Social Science and Medicine,* **11**, 245–50.

Matthews, W.B. (1985a) Clinical aspects: course and prognosis, in *McAlpine's Multiple Sclerosis* (eds W.B. Matthews, E.D. Acheson, J.R. Batchelor and R.O. Weller). Churchill Livingstone, London, pp. 49–72.

Matthews, W.B. (1985b) Symptoms and signs, in *McAlpine's Multiple Sclerosis* (eds W.B. Matthews, E.D. Acheson, J.R. Batchelor and R.O. Weller). Churchill Livingstone, London, pp. 96–145.

Pollock, K. (1984) Mind and Matter. Ph.D. thesis University of Cambridge.

Poskanzer, D.L., Prenney, L.B., Sheridan, J.L. *et al.* (1980) Multiple sclerosis in the Orkney and Shetland Islands. 1. Epidemiology, clinical factors, and methodology. *Journal of Epidemiology and Community Health,* **34**, 229–39.

Power, P.W. (1985) Family coping behaviours in chronic illness: a rehabilitation perspective. *Rehabilitation Literature,* **46**, 78–83.

Robinson, I. (1988a) Managing symptoms in chronic disease: some dimensions of patients' experience. *International Disability Studies,* **1**, 112–18.

Robinson, I. (1988b) *Multiple Sclerosis.* Routledge, London.

Robinson, I. (1988c) Reconstructing lives: managing lives with multiple sclerosis, in *Living with Chronic Illness* (eds R. Anderson and M. Bury). Unwin Hyman, London.

Sackett, D.L. and Snow, J.C. (1979) The magnitude and measurement of compliance, in *Compliance in Health Care* (eds R.B. Haynes, D.W. Taylor and D.L. Sackett). John Hopkins University Press, Baltimore.

Stewart, D.C. and Sullivan, T.J. (1982) Illness behaviour and the sick role: the case of multiple sclerosis. *Social Science and Medicine,* **16**, 1397–404.

Stone, G. (1979) Patient compliance and the role of the expert. *Journal of Social Issues,* **35**, 34–59.

Thompson, J. (1984a) Compliance, in *The Experience of Illness* (R. Fitzpatrick, J. Hinton, S. Newman *et al.*). Tavistock, London, pp. 109–31.

Thompson, J. (1984b) Communicating with patients, in *The Experience of Illness* (R. Fitzpatrick, J. Hinton, S. Newman *et al.*). Tavistock, London, pp. 87–108)

Thompson, M.I. and Haran, D. (1984) Living with amputation: what it means for patients and their helpers. *International Journal of Rehabilitation Research,* **7**, 283–92.

Tuckett, D., Boulton, M., Olson, C. *et al.* (1985) *Meetings Between Experts.* Tavistock, London.

Tyerman, A. and Humphrey, M. (1984) Changes in self concept following severe head injury. *International Journal of Rehabilitation Research,* **7**, 11–23.

2

Multiple sclerosis: Neurology

Leo S. Lange

There is still no consensus on the cause of this common disabling disease. The available evidence suggests that there may be an inborn susceptibility combined with some environmental precipitating factor which damages the central nervous system (CNS).

The illness usually affects young people initially, the common age of first symptoms being between 20 and 40 years, and there is a slight preponderance amongst females. Western Europeans and their descendants are most vulnerable, although the disease has been documented in African and Oriental ethnic groups. The prevalence of disease is highest in northern climes, increasing substantially the further north one travels with a reciprocal distribution in the southern hemisphere (Swingler and Compston, 1986; Skegg et al., 1987). Migration studies from low to high risk areas and vice versa suggest that there is an environmental factor in high risk regions that acts to precipitate the illness, and that the susceptibility is already established by the age of puberty or thereabouts (Alter et al., 1978). There have been thoroughly researched clusters of disease; the best known is probably the 'epidemic' of MS in the Faroes in the 20 years following World War II attributed to the billeting of British troops and their impedimenta on the islands in 1943 (Kurtzke and Hyllested, 1975).

The view that there was an epidemic of MS has been recently challenged and a genetic basis for the geographical distribution postulated, raising doubts about the presence of a potent environmental factor (Poser et al., 1988).

An infective aetiology has been sought for many years and there is evidence for the presence of an active immunological response in MS. Elevated levels of antibody to a number of different viruses have been detected in the cerebrospinal fluid (CSF) and there is good reason to believe that the antibody is elaborated within the nervous system, and has not just leaked into it from the blood (Norrby,

1978). No consistent virus isolations have been achieved and shown to be causally relevant.

The pathological abnormality in MS is an area in which the myelin sheathing nerve fibres has been damaged with relative preservation of the axons. The lesions are perivenular and tend to spread along the venules with considerable inflammatory cellular infiltration, the probable source of the antibodies detectable in the CSF. In the later stages gliosis or scarring occurs and the lesion is referred to as a plaque. There is thought to be an initial breakdown of the blood–brain barrier, enabling the inflammatory cells to penetrate into the CNS. The most frequently involved regions are the periventricular white matter in the hemispheres, with lesions commonly appearing in the brainstem, cerebellum, optic nerves and spinal cord.

Twin studies lend support to theories which postulate the relevance of both genetic and environmental factors in the aetiology (Ebers *et al.*, 1986). Human leukocyte antigen (HLA) studies have shown an increased prevalence of certain factors, notably Dr2, amongst patients with MS, adding weight to the suggestion of a genetic factor in the aetiology (Francis *et al.*, 1987). The risk of developing the disease is also slightly increased for first-degree relatives.

The severity of illness varies enormously and unpredictably within and between patients with few reliable indicators to the prognosis. Estimates of the incidence of disease probably err on the low side as many cases which are mild or benign infection may never come to light, and there are authenticated reports of the lesions of MS at autopsy in subjects who had been neurologically asymptomatic. As many as one in four of all patients may have occasional attacks of disease without any lasting disability, and may lead an entirely normal life without any limitations. Of the others a number progress rapidly to a stage of profound incapacity within a period of months or a few years and the remainder will suffer intermittent or progressive disablement over decades with possible shortening of the life span. Acute episodes of neurological disturbance characteristically evolve over a matter of days, and recover over some weeks, but short-lived symptoms are not uncommon, and often in the later stages progressive neurological disability may supervene on a previously episodic course. In some patients the demyelinating process appears to be steadily progressive from the outset.

SYMPTOMS AND SIGNS

The clinical manifestations will depend upon the anatomical site affected by demyelination. If the optic nerve is involved, pain is often felt in the eye for a few days prior to the onset of visual blurring which may then worsen over some days before starting to recover. Return of central vision may take some weeks, and is often complete. A lesion in the brainstem may produce vertigo, imbalance, incoordination, dysarthria, diplopia, dysphagia, facial numbness or pain, limb weakness and sensory impairment. How many of these features are present will depend upon the size and multiplicity of lesions. Cervical spinal cord lesions often present with loss of sensation in the arm producing severe ataxia and, if appropriate tracts are affected, weakness and sensory loss in both legs with loss of sphincter control. Epilepsy, either focal or generalized, may occur, and intellectual functions may be impaired with alteration of personality when there are plaques in the cerebral hemispheres. Evidence of focal damage such as dysphasia may be present. In addition to the symptoms which can easily be related to anatomical sites, many patients will describe feeling exhausted and depressed prior to a relapse.

Neurological examination in the vast majority of instances will reveal physical signs appropriate to the patient's complaints. Very occasionally special investigations will reveal abnormalities when there is no clinically detectable impairment of function. Great care must then be exercised to evaluate the patient's symptoms in the light of these findings, as the mere presence of abnormalities is no guide to their clinical relevance.

Dysarthria, dysphasia or intellectual impairment may be obvious on taking the history. Visual acuity may be impaired and the pupil may constrict only sluggishly to direct illumination in patients with optic neuritis. In the acute stage the optic disc may appear to be normal, or swollen if the plaque is close to the optic nerve head, and after some weeks the disc generally pales. A visual field defect may be present, either a monocular scotoma, or an homonymous one depicting a visual tract or radiation lesion. Abnormalities of ocular movement accompany diplopia, and nystagmus is often seen with lesions in the vestibulo-cerebellar connections associated with limb ataxia and impaired balance.

Loss of power in the limbs is usually accompanied by increased muscle tone and spasticity may generate muscle spasms. Loss of proprioceptive input from lesions in the posterior columns of the spinal cord will produce sensory ataxia and 'uselessness' of the affected limb, with objective evidence of sensory loss. The deep tendon reflexes may be brisk and plantar responses extensor when the corticospinal tract is affected.

INVESTIGATION

The diagnosis of MS rests on the presence of multiple lesions within the white matter of the CNS which have appeared over a time span of at least six months in the absence of any cause other than demyelination.

Haematology and biochemistry are essential to exclude anaemia, polycythaemia, metabolic disorders and system (collagen) disorders.

Chest X-ray should be carried out where appropriate to exclude neoplasia, tuberculosis and sarcoidosis.

Electrical evoked responses may be carried out to test the integrity of the conducting pathways in the CNS, and magnetic stimulation of the cerebral cortex provides information about the motor pathways.

Computerized tomographic brain scanning may show atrophy of the cerebral or cerebellar substance and with large doses of intravenous contrast medium may show up areas of demyelination.

Magnetic resonance imaging (MRI) of the brain, however, is the most reliable method of demonstrating the presence of lesions and opens up possibilities of measuring quantitatively the amount of damaged brain in serial studies. This will be invaluable in assessment of any form of therapy as an adjunct to clinical evaluation. The mere presence of lesions does not, however, confirm a diagnosis of MS as many other conditions may produce similar effects.

Examination of the CSF may confirm the presence of immunoglobulin (IgG) and electrophoresis may show the IgG to be oligoclonal, in bands present in CSF and not serum, confirming its CNS origin.

MANAGEMENT

Patients presenting to doctors with neurological symptoms are concerned about their disability, anxious about the cause of the trouble and its implications, and seek therapy. Members of a well-informed public who experience symptoms of a common disease may well be acquainted with sufferers from the disease and jump to unwarranted diagnostic conclusions. When the nervous system responds to any insult, be it trauma, tumour, demyelination, infection or toxin, it does so by producing symptoms which usually indicate only the anatomical site of the lesion. Thus, although MS may produce tingling sensations, so may pressure on a peripheral nerve caused, for instance, by leaning on the elbow, or focal sensory epilepsy due to a cerebral tumour.

The doctor's first duty is to try to establish a diagnosis. It may be possible to do so purely on the basis of the history and clinical features, but often further investigation will be necessary. There is, however, still no test which will confirm the diagnosis of MS or refute it categorically, and the final decision will rest on the physician's analysis of the clinical and laboratory data. The extent of special investigation will have to be assessed for each individual, taking into account the availability of resources and the amount and value of information likely to be gleaned from the studies.

If the diagnosis is certain and there is no compelling reason to withhold information, the patient should be told with compassion, and with an honest discussion of the possible prognosis. The substantial chance of a benign outlook is worthwhile emphasizing in lightly affected patients. Revelations are often not fully understood or appreciated at the first telling, and it is not unusual to have to go over the whole exposition again at a later date with a member of the family present.

If the diagnosis of MS is in doubt and the patient is not aware of the possibility, there is little to be gained by mentioning it.

Although acute attacks may subside completely without leaving any disability, it is often rewarding to try to hasten recovery with the use of steroid therapy. The mechanism of action of these hormones is not understood but they do appear to lessen morbidity although repeated courses tend to have less effect and ultimately patients may be totally unresponsive. Recent work indicates that very short bursts of high-dosage steroid intravenously may be as good as more prolonged lower dose therapy which runs a much greater risk of undesirable side-effects (Milligan, Newcombe and Compston, 1987). Steroids are immunosuppressive and also have a beneficial effect on cerebral oedema, and the mode of action may involve either of these mechanisms or some other as yet unclear pathway.

As the neurological damage in MS is thought to be due to inappropriate and excessive activity of the immune response, different methods of interfering with immune function have been tried, and many patients are being treated with powerful drugs to this end.

Despite the theoretical rationale underlying this therapy, there is as yet no convincing objective evidence that it is effective in the long run, and there are risks entailed in upsetting the immune system.

Patients who are chronically unwell neglect their diet both in quantity and quality. There have been many anecdotal accounts of the value of special diets in MS but none has really stood up to careful investigation. There is certainly, however, a case for a balanced diet with adequate caloric, trace element and vitamin content. There is also evidence from carefully conducted studies that diets rich in polyunsaturated fats are beneficial and it is commonplace to advise patients to take supplements on a regular basis (Fitzgerald *et al.*, 1987). Apart from the observed amelioration of the disease process, the unsaturated oils provide a substrate for myelin repair.

If fatigue and exhaustion are prominent complaints, patients are encouraged to get as much rest as they require. This often throws an additional burden on the rest of the family and it has to be made quite clear to both patient and helpers that the need for rest is therapeutic and not related to idleness or lack of moral fibre.

Physiotherapy is enormously supportive both during recovery from an acute relapse, and also as maintenance, as exercise often produces a sensation of well-being. Expert treatment may also modify spasticity. Many forms of naturopathy are used by patients, and as long as they are not harmful should not be ridiculed as faith may well have healing properties.

Affective disorders are common, and although depression may be resolved by social help and counselling, there is also a place for drug therapy and the need for this should be carefully assessed.

Sphincter problems require careful evaluation and drug therapy, or occasionally surgical procedures are necessary to make life more comfortable.

One of the most disabling symptoms is severe tremor which may make it impossible for patients to do anything for themselves. It is possible to improve tremor by surgically damaging a part of the contralateral thalamus, but on the whole one is reluctant to recommend a destructive procedure in a progressive disorder with the probability of only partial success.

As patients become physically more disabled they may require mechanical aids, such as walking sticks, elbow crutches, frames and eventually possibly a wheelchair. The most severely affected persons may be able to retain a fair amount of independence with the help of special electronic equipment enabling them to make and answer telephone calls, draw curtains, type letters and messages, and control heating, lighting, radio and television, all from the bed.

Research into the mechanisms of immune function and modulation must eventually lead to a more effective understanding of the nature of this distressing condition, and as a result to effective prophylaxis or cure. Promising ideas and studies should continue to receive enthusiastic support.

REFERENCES

Alter, M., Kahana, E. and Loewenson, R. (1978) Migration and risk of multiple sclerosis. *Neurology*, **28**, 1089–93.

Ebers, G.C., Bulman, D.E., Sadovnick, A.D. *et al.* (1986) A population-based study of multiple sclerosis in twins. *New England Journal of Medicine*, **315**, 1638–42.

Fitzgerald, G.E., Simpson, K.E., Harbige, L.S. *et al.* (1987) The effect of nutritional counselling on dietary compliance and disease course in multiple sclerosis patients over three years, in *Multiple Sclerosis: Immunological, diagnostic and therapeutic aspects.* (eds F.C. Rose and R. Jones). John Libbey Pubs., London, pp. 189–99.

Francis, D.A., Compston, D.A.S., Batchelor, J.R. *et al.* (1987) A reassessment of the risk of multiple sclerosis developing in patients with optic neuritis after extended follow-up. *Journal of Neurology, Neurosurgery and Psychiatry*, **50**, 758–65.

Kurtzke, J.F. and Hyllested, K. (1975) Multiple sclerosis: an epidemic disease in the Faroes. *Transactions of the American Neurological Association*, **100**, 213–15.

Milligan, N.M., Newcombe, R. and Compston, D.A.S. (1987) A double blind controlled trial of high-dose methyl prednisolone in patients with multiple sclerosis. 1. Clinical effects. *Journal of Neurology, Neurosurgery and Psychiatry*, **50**, 511–16.

Norrby, E. (1978) Viral antibodies in multiple sclerosis. *Progress in Medical Virology*, 7, 168–80.

Poser, Ch.M., Hibberd, P.L., Benedikz, J. *et al.* (1988) Analysis of the 'epidemic' of multiple sclerosis in the Faroe Islands. *Neuroepidemilogy*, 7, 168–80.

Skegg, D.C.B., Corwin, P.A., Craven, R.S. *et al.* (1987) Occurrence of multiple sclerosis in the North and South of New Zealand. *Journal of Neurology, Neurosurgery and Psychiatry*, **50**, 137–9.

Swingler, R.J. and Compston, D. (1986) The distribution of multiple sclerosis in the United Kingdom. *Journal of Neurology, Neurosurgery and Psychiatry*, **49**, 1115–24.

FURTHER READING

Clifford Rose, F. and Jones, R. (eds) (1987) *Multiple Sclerosis:*

Immunological, diagnostic and therapeutic aspects. John Libbey, London.

Matthews, W.B., Acheson, E.D., Batchelor, J.R. *et al.* (eds) (1985) *McAlpine's Multiple Sclerosis.* Churchill Livingstone, London.

McDonald, W.I. and Silberberg, D.H. (eds) (1986) *Multiple Sclerosis.* Butterworths, London.

Poser, C.M., Paty, D.W., Scheinberg, L. *et al.* (eds) (1984) *The Diagnosis of Multiple Sclerosis.* Thieme-Stratton Inc., New York.

3

A therapeutic approach to management

Lorraine H. De Souza

First encounters between therapists and people with multiple sclerosis (MS) generally occur in some type of crisis situation, and in a variety of settings. Patients may be admitted to hospital for a series of tests to confirm diagnosis, or during an exacerbation needing neuro-medical management. They may be seen in departments of therapy, when new symptoms of MS require treatment, or in special clinics when it is necessary to provide, for instance, continence aids, communication aids or a wheelchair. Sometimes patients are seen in their homes, when adaptations are required to secure independent living. With all such situations, therapeutic intervention deals with the immediate needs of the MS patient to achieve a specific goal of treatment. Having achieved the goal of treatment, the MS patient is then discharged from therapy. This approach to therapeutic intervention is based on an acute care model (see Figure 3.1) and although useful in certain situations, such as the acute exacerbation of MS, if used exclusively it presents therapy as a series of unconnected episodes.

In addition, therapists who only intervene with treatment in crisis situations see the MS patient at their worst; for example, when they are hospitalized during a relapse, or when they are becoming profoundly disabled and need aids and adaptations, such as a wheelchair or catheter.

Many therapists working with the acute care model of treatment in MS may feel that little can be done to effect any long-term benefits from continuing treatment. When they are confronted by a patient with multiple and sometimes severe impairment, therapists tend to identify the deficits, disabilities and handicaps and to devise therapy aimed at reducing and eliminating them. In the case of MS, the majority of such therapeutic strategies will wholly or partially fail, and therapists will be left with negative impressions of MS patients which may accumulate during a professional career.

Figure 3.1 A model for acute care

REFERRAL → ASSESSMENT → INTERVENTION → DISCHARGE
        ↓
RE-REFERRAL

Such negative impressions of people with MS are often reinforced by other professionals who may agree that MS sufferers are 'difficult' patients and will get worse anyway, or by the patient and family who may choose to behave in a negative manner. These attitudes are fostered further by advertising and the media who present negative images of disability in order to fund-raise or further causes.

Current writing on disability and chronic illness has been criticized for focusing on 'problems' and therefore reinforcing negative stereotypes. A more balanced view presenting the ups as well as downs of living with disability has been called for (Shearer, 1981; Oliver, 1983), and it encourages a more positive attitude to consider disablement as just one of a variety of ways in which a normal life may be pursued.

In order to counteract negative attitudes about people with MS, which may be prevalent in workplaces and society at large, therapists need to be confident of factual information available about the disease. It is important to realize that people with MS not only have a near normal life expectancy (Matthews *et al.*, 1985; p.60), but also a normal expectation of life. In addition, only 15–20% become severely disabled (Scheinberg *et al.*, 1984), which implies that the majority will not. Furthermore, people with MS can and do experience life to the full including love, marriage, children, work and happiness.

The role of therapy is to help the person learn to live with MS and to lead the life they choose at each stage of the disease. The therapist therefore cannot just offer treatment, but must also offer the care and support necessary to allow MS patients to make informed choices about their lives and circumstances.

The management of MS therefore involves therapists in assuming several different roles with the amount and type of intervention tailored according to the needs of patients. A therapeutic model for chronic care is the most appropriate, and implies that therapy is ongoing, is planned for long-term care, and is sufficiently flexible to account for the fluctuating nature of the disease (see Figure 3.2).

Figure 3.2 A model for chronic care

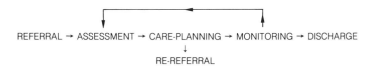

REFERRAL → ASSESSMENT → CARE-PLANNING → MONITORING → DISCHARGE
↓
RE-REFERRAL

ADVANTAGES OF CHRONIC CARE MODEL

With a chronic care model therapists can utilize a wide range of their skills and knowledge, not only to treat MS patients within the scope of their own profession, but also to extend the help for patients by referring to other professionals as appropriate. A system of regular review and evaluation ensures that the patient's condition is monitored. In this way therapists can determine if abilities are being maximized by the patient, and ensure that the commencement of new symptoms are identified at the earliest opportunity.

Therapists have the opportunity to work with patients during periods of remission, when the MS is more stable and the patient feels relatively well. During these periods there is a better chance that treatment can result in real gains in ability. The long-term nature of the chronic care model allows professionals gradually to introduce preventative therapeutic regimens in order to minimize the development and occurrence of common complications in MS, such as contractures and pressure sores.

Regular case review opens up networks of communication between the various disciplines involved in the management of people with MS. By forging such links within the team of professional carers a more coordinated approach can be achieved. This will ensure that the person with MS, and the family, are not overloaded with therapies and advice at some times, while being left with none at all at other times. Discussion of treatments and aims of therapy by the various professionals involved will ensure that there is some consistency in the advice given to the patient and family. In addition, it is important that all the team members are aware of what treatment is being implemented at any one time. This will ensure that the treatment being used by one professional does not conflict with that being given by another. If good coordination of care is implemented, professionals can adopt strategies which enhance and reinforce each other's treatment. This type of approach fosters the confidence of the patient and family, as the same messages are given to them by the various team members.

Finally, by working with a model of chronic care, therapists and other health carers can use their skills to help people with MS and their families to prepare physically and emotionally for life events. Planning and preparation with professional advice and guidance in advance will help MS patients cope with events such as pregnancy and childbirth, starting work, getting a wheelchair, or extending leisure opportunities for those who become unemployed.

CONCEPTS OF CHRONIC CARE

Although different professional carers may have varying amounts of involvement in patient management at various stages of the disease, the team should define some basic concepts to follow. Ashburn and De Souza (1988) have suggested the following concepts which should be integrated into plans of treatment:

1. Long-term management is essential in a long-term disease such as MS. Short-term management programmes are inadequate and frequently lead to an *ad hoc* supportive process instead of a determined plan to improve or maintain function of an individual. The long-term plan for treatment should consist of a programme of continuing involvement with varied intensity throughout a patient's life. Regular input from professionals will need to change appropriately, with the amount of treatment offered tailored to the varying fluctuations of the disease.
2. Early referral is desirable in order to commence appropriate management. A therapy such as diet has preventative elements and nutritional advice needs to be given early. Others such as physiotherapy are frequently only instigated when disabilities are well established. Such late referrals neglect the fact that advice or treatment given in time can often prevent a symptom from developing into a handicap.
3. Regular assessments allow early identification of new symptoms or changes in existing symptoms, for example, the development of pressure sores. Early identification facilitates early treatment and may prevent periods of incapacity and even hospitalization. In addition, regular assessments provide a complete and accurate history of the progression of MS in individual patients. For the patient, regular assessments also provide support and encouragement for the therapeutic strategies already initiated.

27

4. A positive attitude by therapists should try to emphasize abilities and achievements rather than disabilities and handicaps. Even maintaining a functional level should be identified as a positive achievement. The effect of expectation on performance is a vital contributing element in any management programme and, accordingly, a feeling of success at achieving the best level of function possible at each stage of the disease should be encouraged for each individual patient.

5. Correct information should be presented accurately and in an unambiguous manner in order to help the MS patient understand the disease and how his body reacts to it. When giving reassurance to patients therapists must avoid fostering false hopes. Many patients acquire information about their disease which is misleading and part of the supportive role of the therapist is to discover their level of knowledge and to help them to advance it as necessary.

6. Patient responsibility involves fostering a self-help attitude to treatment. This underlines the fact that the patients are not passive recipients of care but are actively involved and responsible in their own management programme and the decision-making processes. Equally the patient needs to understand the role of the therapists and the possible benefits of their professional skills. Patients may be unable to acknowledge or undertake such responsibilities, and for these, counselling may be appropriate.

7. Continuity of care for the individual patient should be ensured between all the professionals involved in the management programme. This fosters in the patient a feeling of confidence in those involved in his case and hence a more positive attitude to his treatment. This is preferable to the negative attitude that can arise when the patient feels he is being 'pillar-to-posted' around the services. Each professional can play a part by ensuring that the results of assessments, aims, objectives and reports of treatment are available between in-patient, out-patient and community services.

8. Team work relies on accurate and regular communication between team members, including the person with MS, their family and carers.

9. A total over-view of each patient's management can only be achieved if the professionals themselves have a sound knowledge of the condition and the factors influencing it. Areas of management often neglected or overlooked are limitations of social interaction caused by disability. Reactions of family members,

friends or work colleagues must be taken into account when therapeutic intervention is initiated. Changes made too drastically can disrupt a patient's life style unexpectedly and cause more problems than they solve. It is therefore necessary to gear treatment to each individual person with MS within the context of a home and social life, and the opportunities available for work and leisure activities. Each member of the management team, including the patient and his/her family, have their role to play in the long-term plan of care.

MS, however, does not run a predictable course, nor a smooth one. Neither does it preclude the development of other illnesses and diseases. The fluctuating nature of MS, interspersed with other unrelated episodes of ill-health, can present a confusing picture in long-term management. As the major part of the management of MS takes place in the community, rather than in hospital, it is the general medical practitioner (GP) who is the key professional in the care of these patients.

THE GENERAL MEDICAL PRACTITIONER

When people feel unwell they usually first consult their GP. In the case of MS, early symptoms may suggest a number of diseases, only one of which may be MS. Where there has been only a single episode which often resolves relatively quickly, MS cannot be suspected, but with evidence of multiple episodes of neurological dysfunction, the GP may refer the patient to a consultant for diagnostic tests.

The 'average' GP can be expected to have approximately one or two MS patients in a practice caseload averaging 2500 at any one time (Hewer, 1980). Therefore, it is unrealistic to assume that GPs will know all about the long-term care and management of MS. Yet patients' expectations of what their doctors can do to help are often very high (A. Burnfield, 1985). Robinson (1987) discusses the pros and cons of the doctor–patient partnership in terms of the different knowledge and experiences each party may bring to the relationship.

Broome and McMullan (1977) have described the role of the GP in the management of physically disabled patients as being:

1. early treatment of disease and help with practical problems;
2. supervision of continuing treatment;

3. coordination of help in the community;
4. personal support to patients and helpers.

The importance of early intervention and continuing clinical involvement in the symptomatic management of MS cannot be underestimated. Bauer (1978) comments that 'improvement in prognosis can be attributed to better symptomatic therapy and more effective management of complications'. This process also involves the prompt prescription of drugs which may alleviate symptoms, and the necessary monitoring of dosage (Matthews *et al.*, 1985; pp. 235–78).

In supervising continuing treatment, the GP can ensure continuity, and a smooth transition, between the hospital regimen and community care. In order to effect some aspects of this, referral to the community nurse or community-based therapists may be appropriate. Gaining access for patients to the therapy professions and the support network largely relies on the willingness of GPs to refer patients. Yet large numbers of MS patients do not appear to be involved with social and therapeutic services (Elian and Dean, 1983; De Souza, 1983).

Ideally, the work of the remedial professionals should be coordinated, and the GP should be sufficiently well informed to help. Mutual cooperation among the professionals involved may also provide mutual learning of each other's roles and abilities to foster discussion of difficult cases from all points of view. The GP should be aware of local variations in what is available, to press for services which are unavailable, and to negotiate for improvements in community care (Broome and McMullan, 1977).

Often the GP will be drawn into discussions with the MS patient and family where advice and help are sought on a number of issues. Some may be directly related to the effects of MS on personal and family life. An example is sexual problems. Here the GP needs to conduct a sensitive and sympathetic consultation in order to determine sexual dysfunction due to the MS, and that which is due to anxiety, fear or fatigue (P. Burnfield, 1978).

Patients may wish to discuss the pros and cons of having children, the effect of pregnancy on the MS, and whether or not their children will develop the disease (Chapter 11). The GP, as the family doctor, is in a position to give the facts required and to facilitate discussion in order to help the couple make their decisions. Subsequently the GP may have to manage the pregnancy of a woman with MS, and knowledge of the individual's case will help the obstetrics team to make their decisions about management for delivery and post-natal care.

The MS patient, a family member, or the professional carers may complain to the doctor of depression. Sometimes depression prevents activities such as those required for daily living, or those necessary for implementing therapeutic programmes. The GP should be aware that some depression is a result of grief, and is a normal reaction to physical dysfunction. However, other states of depression, which may be due to the MS, or due to another unrelated factor, can become an affective disorder. Stewart and Shields (1983) discuss the assessment and management of grief in chronic illness, and describe the diagnosis and differential diagnosis of grief and depression.

Responsibility for the treatment of symptoms, and long-term medical management of MS patients, are generally undertaken by the GP. This approach should not be avoided because, as Bauer (1978; p.8) writes:

> . . . it is based on the keener realisation that, beyond the pathologic condition, we are dealing with the destinies, the fortunes, and the concerns of persons afflicted by MS over many years, quite often a major part of their lifespan.

CHOICES FOR TREATMENT

The treatments, advice or interventions offered to MS patients by the various professionals involved in their care form only some aspects of all the advice or help that is offered on how to cope with MS (see Figure 3.3). Some of the influences, for example media articles, may hold more sway with an individual with MS than even the best professional advice. It is important for the professional carers to recognize that, in the face of a progressive and incurable disease, MS patients may need to explore all the possibilities offered to help them cope. An understanding of this need is called for, and part of the professionals' work may be to help MS patients rationalize their expectations of new treatments. This may involve the professional in finding out details of treatments, and explaining the evidence for and against to the MS patient.

Often the patient seeks the professional's advice about treatments. Such consultation should be encouraged in order to generate discussion, and the professional should be wary of ridiculing new treatments, no matter how unlikely they may seem. At the same

Figure 3.3 An example of the diverse sources of information which may influence life-style of the MS patient. The professional sources are in italics

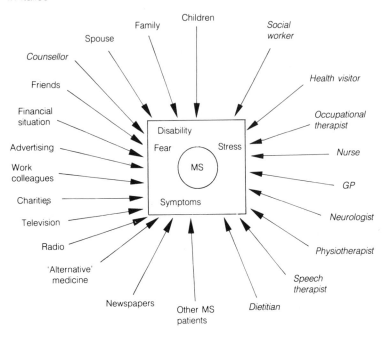

time, professionals have a duty clearly to warn patients about harmful treatments or bogus practitioners. Where the MS patient has trust and confidence in the professional's ability, advice is more often sought and recommendations more readily taken.

Part of the professional's work is to make the therapy treatments and advice given to MS patients understandable and relevant to each individual's circumstances and needs. However, it is not the role of professional carers to control the lives of MS patients. The patients themselves must be allowed to make their own decisions concerning the treatment and management of their MS. Perhaps part of the professional carer's role is to help MS patients preserve their rights of self-determination.

But patients can only exercise this right if they have sufficient knowledge about MS and how it affects them. With sound knowledge and good advice, patients may be able to make informed decisions in order to determine their life styles with MS.

REFERENCES

Ashburn, A. and De Souza, L.H. (1988) An approach to the management of multiple sclerosis. *Physiotherapy Practice,* **4**, 139–45.

Bauer, H.J. (1978) Problems of symptomatic therapy in multiple sclerosis. *Neurology,* **28**, 8–20.

Broome, M. and McMullan, J.J. (1977) Resettlement in the community, in *Rehabilitation Today* (ed. S. Mattingly). Update Publications Ltd., London.

Burnfield, A. (1985) *Multiple Sclerosis: A personal exploration.* Souvenir Press, London.

Burnfield, P. (1978) Sexual problems and multiple sclerosis. *British Journal of Family Planning,* **4**, 2–5.

De Souza, L.H. (1983) Physiotherapy for multiple sclerosis patients. *Lancet,* **i**, 8339; 1444.

Elian, M. and Dean, G. (1983) Need for and use of social and health services by MS patients living at home in England. *Lancet,* **i**, 8339; 1091–3.

Hewer, R.L. (1980) Multiple sclerosis management and rehabilitation. *International Rehabilitation Medicine,* **2**, 116–25.

Matthews, W.B., Acheson, E.D., Batchelor, J.R. *et al.* (eds) (1985) *McAlpine's Multiple Sclerosis.* Churchill Livingstone, London.

Oliver, M.J. (1983) *Social Work With Disabled People.* Macmillan, London.

Robinson, I. (1987) Productive partnership? The profession and the patient in the management of multiple sclerosis, in *Multiple Sclerosis: Immunological, diagnostic and therapeutic aspects* (eds F.C. Rose and R. Jones). John Libbey Publications, London, pp. 245–53.

Scheinberg, L., Kalb, R., Larocca, N. *et al.* (1984) The doctor–patient relationship in multiple sclerosis, in *The Diagnosis of Multiple Sclerosis* (ed. C.M. Poser). Thieme-Stratton Inc., New York, pp. 205–15.

Shearer, A. (1981) *Disability: Whose Handicap?* Basil Blackwell, Oxford.

Stewart, T. and Shields, C.R. (1983) Grief in chronic illness: assessment and management. *Archives of Physical Medicine and Rehabilitation,* **66**, 447–50.

4

Physiotherapy

Lorraine H. De Souza

Abnormalities of movement are often the first outward signs that a person has multiple sclerosis (MS), and the loss of a movement skill, or the ability to perform a functional activity, may be the first indication to a patient or professional that MS is a progressively disabling disease. When motor disability increases to an arbitrary level of handicap, some people with MS may be referred for physiotherapy. By this stage disease has damaged the central nervous system, physical deficits will have created a level of functional impairment, and disabilities secondary to that caused by the MS may have developed.

The loss of normal movement skills not only has a physical effect on the MS patient, but also an often profound psychological effect. While during the early stages of the disease the person may have been relatively fit, and of normal appearance, the first signs of physical impairment will delineate the physical and psychological vulnerability of having MS. Physical abilities previously taken for granted, become unreliable, and patients experience unwelcomed changes in their self-image. The act of seeking help from a physio- therapist is an admission in itself that physical therapy is required, and many patients will not be comfortable with the situation. The therapist may be viewed as a friend who can help the patient to over- come the physical disabilities, or as a foe who could expose further physical weaknesses. Physiotherapists need to be aware that the same professional skills which can help patients improve movement ability can also undermine their self-confidence.

Treating the person with MS requires not only clinical skills, but also a sympathetic approach, a willingness to spend time and to have patience (Hewer, 1980). The abilities of the physiotherapist, in terms of maturity and experience as well as in terms of clinical skills, play the greatest role in determining the success or failure of treatment. Successful treatment cannot be measured by whether or not the MS patient improves, but rather by whether or not the best level of activity is achieved with respect to an individual's life style at each stage of the disease.

THERAPEUTIC ROLES

The rehabilitative role is the one most commonly identified by other professionals, and by physiotherapists themselves, as being the essential role in the treatment of MS patients. The redressing and retraining of postural and movement disorders caused by MS constitutes the major work of the physiotherapist in this field. However, a rehabilitative role is not always the most appropriate one to assume, and is rarely exclusively used.

Because of the progressive nature of the disease a preventative therapeutic role is important. However, as there is no prognosis for any individual case of MS, a sensible approach is called for. Physiotherapists should avoid either consciously or sub-consciously instilling fear in patients of what may happen in the future, yet should not fight shy of issues necessary to implementing preventative treatments where appropriate.

A supportive role is often the one most appropriate to adopt when active treatment is inappropriate. Situations such as an acute relapse call for the physiotherapist to implement maintenance regimens which are often passive in nature. A supportive approach in such situations can help to dispel patients' fears that the physiotherapist is only interested in them when they are well, and does not offer help or contact when they get worse.

People with MS will often seek advice from the physiotherapist on many subjects, while therapists will give advice to patients both formally and informally. In assuming an advisory role the physiotherapist should be quite clear what constitutes professional advice for which she has training and clinical experience to give, and which does not, and the patient needs to be made aware of the difference.

Health education is an important adjunct to treatment. The physiotherapist has his/her role to play in helping patients understand how the MS affects their bodies. For each individual patient an understanding of the comparative values of exercise and activity, and rest, relaxation and recuperation, will add to knowledge for developing coping strategies in everyday life.

To deal successfully with MS patients, the physiotherapist needs to be versatile and intuitive in order to assume different roles, or mix roles, appropriately. A wide range of clinical skills are called into play in the flexible approach to treatment required for this complex condition. A strict neurodevelopmental approach is largely redundant in the treatment of MS, as the degenerative nature of the disease is a reverse of the theoretical assumptions of this type of approach (Bobath, 1978). The physiotherapist needs to be able and competent to change the direction and approach to treatment in response to new conditions presented by the fluctuations and progression of MS.

PRINCIPLES OF PHYSIOTHERAPY

The management of MS patients by physiotherapists should be viewed and planned on a long-term rather than a short-term basis. Early referral is essential for planning a long-term management programme, and for instigating preventative therapeutic regimens. Short-term treatment programmes are inadequate in the care of MS patients and often leads to an *ad hoc* supportive process instead of a determined plan to maintain or improve functional movement in an individual. A continuing involvement provides regular input from the physiotherapist with the amount and type of treatment offered varying in intensity and tailored to the fluctuations of the disease (Ashburn and De Souza, 1988).

The principles of treatment are:

1. To encourage the development of strategies of movement;
2. to encourage the learning of motor skills;
3. to improve the quality of patterns of movement;
4. to minimize abnormalities of muscle tone;
5. to emphasize the functional application of physiotherapy;
6. to support the patient in order to maintain motivation and cooperation, and to reinforce therapy;
7. to implement preventative therapy;
8. to educate the person towards a greater understanding of the symptoms of MS and how they affect activities of daily living.

Although each MS person is an individual, and must be treated as such, four primary aims of physiotherapy treatment have been identified (Ashburn and De Souza, 1988):

1. To maintain and increase range of movement;
2. to encourage postural stability;

3. to prevent contractures;
4. to maintain and encourage weight-bearing.

ASSESSMENT AND PLANNING OF TREATMENT

Physiotherapy treatment programmes must be tailored to each individual on the basis of accurate and detailed assessment. Graded objective assessments of sensorimotor function of upper and lower limbs, functional movements and daily living activities should be routinely recorded and kept as a documentation of a patient's progression and response to therapy. The motor deficits contributing to altered function should be identified and in turn used to indicate the priorities for treatment.

Special care should be taken to identify complications such as contractures and deformities, atrophy, reduced mobility, loss of movement awareness and sensory deprivation which occur in MS simply from disuse.

Goal-orientated treatment programmes may be decided on the basis of assessment. The main deficits of motor control causing abnormalities of posture, balance, muscle tone and coordination of movement will require redressing through physiotherapy programmes. However, all regimens requiring active exercises should take into account the fatigue levels of the MS patient.

Re-assessment at regular intervals ensures that changing symptoms, gains achieved and progression of the disease are adjusted for in treatment programmes. Formal documentation in the medical records of all physiotherapeutic evaluations provides a concrete history of the sensorimotor symptomology and treatment of each patient. Each assessment should conclude with a clear statement of the aims of treatment for that stage, and each subsequent assessment should evaluate how far the aims have been fulfilled.

Part of each assessment should include a self evaluation by the person with MS. Such an exercise has several purposes. The physiotherapist obtains valuable information on how the patient views his own abilities and disabilities, and by asking the patient to prioritize, the therapist becomes aware of which areas are seen as more important than others. Often the patient's priorities are different from the therapist's, and further discussion will need to take place so that both therapist and patient agree to a treatment programme with both parties working together to achieve the same goals. Therapists can ascertain patients' expectations of treatment and, where appropriate, modify those expectations by explanation and discussion. By this process patients gain some insight into the effects of MS on sensorimotor function, and can be encouraged by the physiotherapist to analyse these effects with respect to their own life styles. Patients will also gain some knowledge of what physiotherapy has to offer, and therefore when to seek advice and treatment from a physiotherapist.

Physiotherapy assessments, however, do not provide the solutions to the problem of treatment for people with MS. Assessment is merely a clinical tool used by the physiotherapist to gain detailed insight into the patient's condition and functional status. The power of this tool lies in the ability of the therapist to interpret the assessment, and use the information to formulate a relevant and workable plan of treatment.

IDENTIFICATION OF MOVEMENT DEFICITS AND AIMS OF TREATMENT

When planning treatment programmes there are five key areas of sensorimotor function which need to be considered. These key areas form a basis for the re-education of movement, and the type of physiotherapy techniques which will be used.

Posture

The main postural abnormalities which can occur in MS are unilateral or bilateral flexion of the hips, an exaggerated lumbar lordosis of the spine, stooped shoulders, unilateral or bilateral hyperextension of the knee, and the loss of trunk rotation on movement.

Adequate daily stretching of affected muscle groups will help to prevent postural abnormalities from becoming fixed and limiting movement. Encouraging postural awareness will help the MS patient to recognize good posture in sitting and or standing, and to learn how to correct poor posture in these positions. The use of reflex-inhibiting patterns will help to prevent the development of spastic contractures (Bobath, 1978), which, in turn, reduces the possibility of pressure sores.

Balance

It is necessary to determine whether or not balance and save reactions are normal, reduced or absent. Assessment in both static postures and during movement should be carried out as part of the clinical evaluation. Maintaining equilibrium relies not only on the functional integrity of the vestibular apparatus, but also on sensory input from proprioceptors and pressure receptors. Therefore a sensory assessment may be necessary. The emphasis of treatment should be to encourage movements and functional activities, such as transfers, which will facilitate and stimulate balance reactions. Motor control of the head and trunk is the key to maintaining stability in both static postures and during movement. The key points of movement are proximal, and co-contraction at the proximal joints aids stability of the limb girdles on the body axis.

Muscle tone

Tone may be abnormally increased or decreased in muscle groups, but many MS patients may show tone abnormalities in both directions. There are four important components to the management of spasticity (Todd, 1982):

1. Education of the need to avoid positions and activities that increase tone or reinforce abnormal movement patterns;
2. daily walking, or standing for weight bearing;
3. regular stretching of hypertonic muscle groups;
4. avoidance of pressure sores, constipation and bladder infections.

Flaccidity is commonly present with both spasticity and ataxia, and treatment strategies need to be used with care in order not to exacerbate other symptoms of MS. Techniques of facilitation are useful, as are movements and postures which load the limb in reflex inhibiting weight-bearing positions. For the purposes of effective treatment, flaccidity should be differentiated from muscle weakness.

Coordination and ataxia

Ataxia is a specific disturbance of motor function which results in loss of coordination and voluntary movements. It is a disturbance

39

which, independently to motor weakness, alters direction and extent of movement and impairs the sustained voluntary and reflex muscle contractions necessary for maintaining posture and equilibrium (Bouillaud, 1846). Lesions of the cerebellum are thought to be most commonly, though not exclusively, to blame. Treating the ataxic MS patient is difficult as these, more than patients with other types of predominant motor symptoms, tend to fluctuate the most. Treatment should be directed at regaining postural stability, and voluntary control of the body's centre of gravity in weight-bearing positions, and weight-transferring movements. A correct body alignment of head and trunk in static postures and during movement should be encouraged, and the re-education of proximal limb muscle groups to stabilize the limb girdles by co-contraction is required. Frenkel's exercises (1890) may be useful for some patients where sensory deficits are not too great.

Fatigue

The management of fatigue should be integrated into physiotherapy programmes by educating patients on the need to pace activities and conserve energy, and on the value of rest. Relaxation regimens can help those who find it difficult to rest, and those who are anxious or in stressful situations. Carefully staged exercise programmes can be used to increase stamina and endurance, but these must be monitored by the therapist. Dietary advice can ensure sufficient caloric intake for needs, and can establish a suitable eating pattern and referral to a dietitian may be necessary (see Chapter 8). The daily pattern of fatigue for each patient should be identified by the physiotherapist in order to give relevant advice, and to plan treatment regimens and home exercise programmes.

The aims of treatment, both for short-term and long-term goals, should indicate a plan of physiotherapy which includes the five areas described above in a coordinated programme of movement re-education.

RE-EDUCATION OF MOVEMENT

Characteristically, the problems of motor control in MS are diverse and often motor symptoms are masked or overlaid by others, producing a confused and conflicting picture of movement disorder.

Detailed physiotherapy assessment will identify the deficits of motor control caused by abnormalities of posture, balance, muscle tone and coordination of movement.

An approach to treatment based on the learning or re-learning of strategies of movement (Carr and Shepherd, 1987) is probably the most relevant for a chronic condition such as MS.

The theory

Learning and adaptation to change are features of all vertebrate central nervous systems and are most highly developed in primates, particularly in humans. The neural mechanisms of learning remain debatable, but evidence from animal experiments suggests that some structural changes occur in parts of the central nervous system (CNS) and in particular at synapses (Raisman and Field, 1973; Wall, 1980).

Several studies show that similar plastic changes in the CNS occur in humans (Bach-y-Rita, 1980). Such structural changes may be similar to those thought to occur when a new motor skill is acquired (Globus *et al.*, 1973; Greenough, 1976). However, an approach to physiotherapy which incorporates learning new motor skills needs numerous repetitions of the movement patterns and therefore requires a good degree of motivation by the patient (De Souza, 1983). To maintain motivation, the exercises set should be functionally orientated to the patient's real world, i.e. to the activities of daily living. In addition, education of the patient to explain and show the relevance of exercises increases his knowledge of the physical management of his disease. The use of education as an adjunct to behavioural therapy is considered to be valuable in the management of chronic disease (Mazzuca, 1982).

As in all learning processes, periods of motor learning are followed by periods of consolidation of the newly acquired knowledge. During consolidation periods patients appear to be making no new progress in therapy. In our experience with MS patients, such periods of no progress can be used in therapy both to recapitulate movements which have already been learnt and also as revision periods for newly acquired motor skills. Therefore, when MS patients show no new progress in therapy, the reinforcement and consolidation of preceding therapy is indicated, and not, as so often occurs, the discontinuation of therapy. The periods of motor learning and of consolidation vary greatly in MS patients but appear to depend generally on age and duration of the disease (De Souza, 1984).

In order to learn the correct force, direction and timing of a pattern of movement, the whole motion must be practised. Correction of inaccuracies and timing of parts of the pattern can be made by the therapist and learnt by the patient as part of the whole movement skill. This approach is much easier and more relevant for the patient to learn than one teaching several component parts of a movement pattern which must then be reassembled in the correct spatial and temporal sequence for functional use (Jones, 1974).

The treatment

Treatment sessions are used to teach patients the appropriate exercises and methods of movement control which will inhibit and counteract the adverse symptoms of multiple sclerosis. Motor control is taught on the basis that only voluntary movement and effort can result in learning, or relearning, of movement strategies. Active-assisted movements are used with grossly disabled patients with the physiotherapist providing the minimum amount of physical contact necessary (De Souza, 1984).

The physiotherapist makes and maintains close contact with the patient, using skills of the voice (Gardiner, 1976) rather than skills of the hands. In this way, as control of movement is learnt by the patient it is seen as a product of the patient's own efforts, rather than a product of the physiotherapist's manipulative skills. This realization is extremely important as the patient is expected to comply with a home regimen of exercises. It is emphasized that practice makes perfect, and daily home exercises are required. The patient is given written exercises and movements to practise at home and these must be achieved in the absence of the physiotherapist. The patient learns to depend on himself for 'treatment', rather than on the physiotherapist. Home regimens are always set at a level which the patient has achieved in a class, therefore he is confident of his own knowledge and ability. Progression of treatment occurs in the class before being included in a home regimen. The physiotherapist checks that home regimens are correctly executed by the patient, and altered if disease symptoms change. She also ensures that the correct balance of different types of exercises is retained (De Souza, 1984).

As exercises, positions or strategies of movement are taught in classes an explanation is always given by the physiotherapist about their relevance for everyday activities. Therefore the patient learns both the voluntary manoeuvre and the purpose for practising it. Reinforcement of both is continual in the class situation. Eventually patients learn to choose appropriate manoeuvres from their repertoire to match the fluctuating day-to-day symptoms of their disease (De Souza, 1984).

A basic exercise programme

An example of a basic exercise programme has been presented by Ashburn and De Souza (1988) and is shown in Figure 4.1. A core set of exercises can be used for different purposes with different MS patients by changing the emphasis of the movement. The emphasis of the movement may be, first, to increase an active range of voluntary control, followed by sustained stretch at the end of the range. Alternatively, the holding of certain postures and positions will encourage stabilization, and can be used for strengthening muscles. Therapists need to communicate to patients that it is the quality of the patterns of movement which are more important than the quantity of repetitions achieved.

A core set of exercises, as shown in the example, are thought to be of general use to most MS patients (Ashburn and De Souza, 1988). However, as no two MS patients will have the same levels of sensorimotor deficits, exercises specific to each individual are required in addition to the basic programme.

MANAGEMENT OF THE PATIENT WITH PREDOMINANTLY SPASTIC SYMPTOMS

The development of spasticity in muscles may, initially, be so slight at first that it may escape the notice of both therapist and patient. Early signs of spasticity being expressed as a symptom of MS may only amount to detecting transient hypertonus in some limb or trunk positions, or the presence of clonus or brisk reflexes on testing. The patient may report intermittent spasms in muscles or just a feeling of tightness or stiffness in a muscle or joint.

Routine assessments should include examination for abnormalities in muscle tone. The physiotherapist generally examines tone by using fast and slow passive movements throughout the normal range of all limb joints. Usually, a qualitative comment of tone records it

43

Figure 4.1 An example of an exercise programme: (1) Knee flexion in prone lying; (2) Hip and knee flexion from supine; (3) Bridging; (4) Knee rolling; (5) Long sitting with arms elevated; (6) Knee flexion with trunk rotation; (7) High kneeling; (8) Standing; (9) Trunk rotation in standing; (10) Hip flexion; (11) Weight transference in step-stride standing; (12) Walking practice.

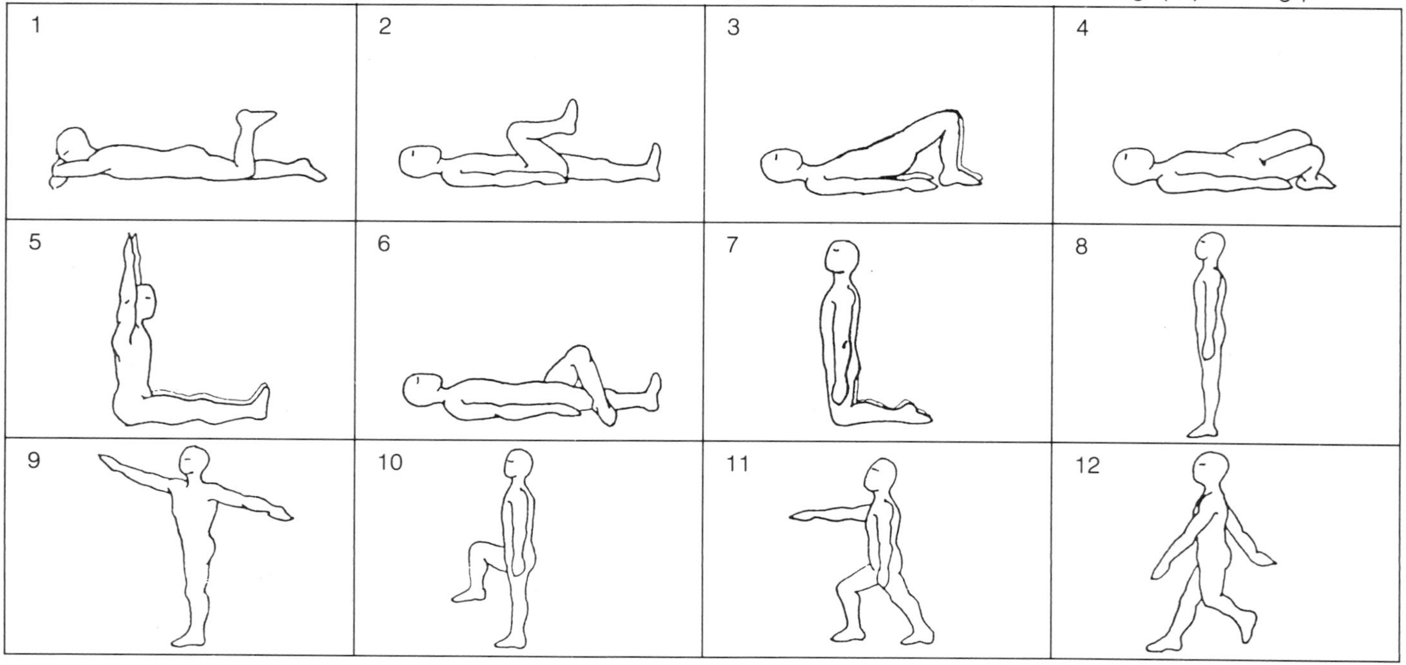

as being abnormally high, abnormally low, or apparently normal. This notation is sufficient for a clinical record and any abnormalities detected should be accompanied by the named muscle groups involved. Sometimes gradings of spasticity, such as the Oswestry Scale (Goff, 1976), may be used, but with these there may be large interobserver variables. The different approaches to the measurement and assessment of spasticity have been reviewed by De Souza and Musa (1987).

The major reason for treating spasticity is to reduce abnormally high muscle tone to a level where residual voluntary movement can be used to best functional effect. By stretching the affected muscles very slowly, and maintaining stretch over a long period of time, spasticity can be reduced and the range of voluntary movement increased (Bobath, 1978; Odeen, 1981). The use of slow stretch of hypertonic muscles can be adapted by employing positions or postures where the affected muscle groups are maintained in a stretched position. These positions are:

1. Prone lying, to stretch the hip flexors;
2. sitting tailor-fashion, to stretch the hip adductors;
3. long sitting, to stretch the knee flexors;
4. side-sitting, to stretch the trunk flexors;
5. standing upright, to stretch the ankle plantiflexors;

The muscle groups mentioned above are those which most commonly show increased tone in MS, and other conditions where there are lesions of the motor pathways in the CNS.

Other techniques, such as cooling the skin over the affected muscle group with ice or cold water (Mead and Knott, 1960), can also effect a temporary reduction in hypertonus. However, when using cold therapy to reduce spasticity in MS patients care should be taken to ensure that adequate circulation to the extremities is present and can be maintained. The use of ice, or cold water, cannot be recommended if the MS patient has noticeably cool lower or upper limb extremities.

Whichever techniques are used, the therapist should have clear reasons for reducing spasticity. The decision to reduce tone, and the amount of reduction aimed for, is only a good decision when more function can be achieved, or management made easier for a carer. In some cases of MS reducing spasticity will uncover other underlying symptoms such as ataxia or muscle weakness, which may be more difficult to control. Some increased tone can be useful to

45

Figure 4.2 Gravity assisted stretch of psoas major by lowering the leg over the side of a low plinth

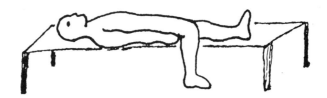

people with MS and may be essential for retaining an ability to walk or transfer. Patients relying on a 'swing to' or 'swing through' gait pattern using crutches, for example, will require a certain level of spasticity in the lower limbs to remain mobile. With these cases, reduction of spasticity should only be attempted if there is a good possibility for retraining a four-point reciprocal gait pattern for which adequate residual voluntary movement is required.

Maintaining standing and weight-bearing for as long as possible is one of the key points in the long-term management of the MS patient. Weight-bearing through the lower limbs is, in itself, a method of controlling the development of abnormally high muscle tone, and is one preventative measure to minimize the possibility of the development of increased tone in the flexor groups of muscles.

The development of flexor spasticity greatly reduces the hope that the patient can continue to be upright and mobile. With these patients the emphasis of treatment needs to be directed at the reduction of flexor muscle tone, the prevention of flexion contractures and, wherever possible, the maintenance of standing transfers.

The muscle most responsible for flexion contractures at the hip is psoas major. Preventative measures to counteract the development of increased tone in psoas should be initiated from the earliest stages of MS by the use of prone lying and by encouraging active contraction of hip extensor muscles using exercise therapy. When a functional contracture is identified, the muscle can be stretched by extending the affected hip passively. This can be achieved with the aid of gravity by lowering the leg over the side of a low plinth (Figure 4.2), or by gentle passive stretch applied manually. In both of these manoeuvres care needs to be taken that the lower lumbar spine remains in a normal lordotic curve. Any sign of 'bowing' in the lumbar region indicates that the muscle is not stretching out, but is simply pulling at the spinal origins. Such an occurrence should be positively avoided as there is a danger of injury to the muscle and the lower lumber spine which could cause unnecessary pain, or instability of the normal articulation of the lumbar vertebrae.

MANAGEMENT OF THE PATIENT WITH PREDOMINANTLY ATAXIC SYMPTOMS

There are several types of ataxias which may be expressed in MS and the neurological assessment and classification of the different types have been described by Morgan (1980).

Observation of ataxic movement, using eye or video recording, show that the symptom manifests itself in movements where groups of muscles are required to act together in varying degrees of co-contraction. The main movement disorders of the ataxic patient are postural instability and the loss of coordination in movement.

In order to retrain postural stability the physiotherapist should direct treatment strategies at encouraging the patient to gain control of the centre of gravity of the body. The unstable ataxic patient generally lowers the centre of gravity by flexing at the hips. In this posture the patient may feel more stable, but is disadvantaged when attempting to walk. In addition, there is a risk of developing functional flexion contractures of the hip. The patient may try to gain further stability by fixing the trunk and locking the knee joints in hyperextension.

To correct this typically abnormal posture the physiotherapist should direct treatment at re-education of the hip extensor muscles first. Later, anterior pelvic tilting should be encouraged. These two exercises may be attempted in a high kneeling position before standing if the patient appears too unstable and fearful of falling.

When the patient has gained some control of hip extension and pelvic rotation, the therapist should progress treatment and re-educate muscle control of inner-range knee movement. Care needs to be taken at this stage to ensure that hip extension and pelvic position is maintained, otherwise the patient's body may 'jack-knife' into flexion at the hips.

To retrain coordination two main areas of movement control should be considered. The first involves the re-education of total body movement patterns and concentrates on control of the head, body axis, and movement of the limb girdles on the body axis. These movements involve the ability to rotate the body around the axis which is used as the internal reference point. By the assessment procedure the physiotherapist will be able to determine the presence

47

or absence of the various body and head righting reflexes (Roberts, 1978), and therefore initiate therapy at the level of impairment identified. Activities which will stimulate these reflexes need to be employed. Rolling from supine to prone, trunk rotations in various positions, turning, and twisting movements all help to re-train the coordination required for the rotatory components of movements. The ability to move the head and trunk segments in a normal temporospatial sequence, and to rotate around the body's axis, is essential for functional movements such as transferring and walking.

The second area of movement control to be considered is that of the re-education of coordination of agonist-antagonist limb muscle groups. The most basic patterns of movements to which therapists should direct treatment are reaching and retrieving in the upper limbs, and gait in the lower limbs. The key points of movement control are proximal, at the shoulder and the hip. The rotator cuff musculature at these joints are anatomically and functionally complex, yet it is the ability of these muscle groups either to stabilize or move the proximal joint appropriately which determines the pattern of movement in the limb.

The coordination of the rotator cuff muscles may be encouraged by active or assisted exercises where the limb passes through arcs of movement, for example, with the upper limb, elevation through shoulder flexion, or elevation through shoulder abduction.

The diagonal arcs of movement may be encouraged by the use of proprioceptive neuro-muscular facilitation (PNF) techniques (Knott and Voss, 1968). However, the main use of manual contact should be to direct the course of movement and, if necessary, to apply some manual resistance to encourage muscle coordination at the proximal joints. The therapist should avoid applying more than the minimum manual resistance appropriate as the MS patient will rapidly fatigue. The physiotherapist may notice that some parts of the arc of movement appear more stable than others. If this is the case, the more stable excursions of the upper limb should be noted as areas on which to attempt to build hand function improvements for activities of daily living such as eating and drinking.

The fluid coordination of agonist-antagonist muscle groups around other limb joints may be encouraged by techniques such as rhythmic stabilizations, rhythmic alternating movements and pendular movement (Gardiner, 1976).

Some authors have suggested the use of weights and weighted cuffs as limb restraints for ataxic patients (Morgan et al., 1975), but point out that these should not be used where weakness is evident.

There appears to be an immediate effect in reducing upper limb ataxia when a weighted cuff is applied (Morgan, 1980), but there is no evidence of any long-term benefit. It is this author's experience that the limb musculature accommodates to the applied weights over a period of time with the ataxia remaining essentially unaltered, and then apparently worsened by the subsequent removal of the weights.

AIDS FOR MOBILITY

The provision of walking aids, such as sticks and crutches, have advantages and disadvantages, which should be considered. Obvious advantages include helping the patient to walk further or faster, or walk with a better gait pattern. With some cases walking aids may increase the patient's stability, or reduce fatigue. For many MS patients, using walking aids can enable them to remain mobile and postpone the necessity to use a wheelchair full time.

The physiotherapist should be aware of the detrimental effects of providing walking aids, and exercise suitable care and precautions in order to minimize them. These detrimental effects are described by Todd (1982). Firstly, the inhibitory effect on spasticity of weight-bearing through the lower limbs will be reduced. Secondly, changes in posture will cause a sideways shift of the trunk if unilateral support is used, or forward trunk flexion with hip flexion when bilateral support is used. Thirdly, as the demand for normal head and trunk movements are lessened, there will be a reduction of balance reactions, which in turn alters muscle tone.

The physiotherapist will need to introduce exercises and activities which will compensate for the inevitable loss of movement ability, and the patient's opportunities of experiencing normal movement.

The detrimental effects described above are further exacerbated if the walking aids are poorly adjusted for an individual patient, and if gait re-education with the walking aid has not been carried out in order to achieve the best gait pattern possible. Apart from the preventative regimens of treatment necessary to counteract the detrimental effects of using walking aids, the physiotherapist will need to implement therapy to maintain mobility and increase strength in the upper limbs. This is particularly important as the MS patient is likely to become progressively more dependent on upper limb support to maintain mobility.

Due to the fluctuating and progressive nature of the disease, the type of walking aid issued to patients should be regularly reviewed.

Follow-up is also necessary if the patient is issued with a walking aid during recovery from relapse. As more voluntary movement is recovered post-relapse, a change in walking aid or use of a different gait pattern may be indicated.

Finally, patients who rely on upper limb support for mobility are often prone to injuries of the muscles, tendons and ligaments, particularly of the shoulders. Such injuries should be treated actively by the physiotherapist when acute, and the development of chronic or recurring injuries avoided wherever possible.

The use of splints and calipers needs to be viewed with the same caution as other walking aids. The therapist should be aware that once a joint is made immobile by a splint or caliper any residual voluntary movement of the joint will be lost, therefore preventative treatment should be initiated. Follow-up is essential to ensure that the orthosis is accurately fitted, and that the patient can don it and use it correctly. Although a splint or caliper may successfully alleviate some mobility problems, other motor symptoms, such as spasticity, may be aggravated. Regular reassessment of the MS patient will help the physiotherapist to identify such occurrences.

When considering giving any aids for mobility the physiotherapist should first assess the MS patient in order to decide on the most suitable type of aid. The use of mobility aids should be incorporated into a plan of long-term management, with short-term goals defined by aims of treatment in specific gait re-eduction programmes.

It is important that the aims, short-term goals and long-term management plan are discussed with the patient and family. Aids for mobility should be introduced with sensitivity as many patients see a stick or crutches as a symbol of their disability, and the need to use a walking aid as a sign that their MS has worsened. The physiotherapist therefore should encourage a positive attitude to the use of walking aids by helping the MS patient to appreciate and experience the advantages of improved mobility.

THE MANAGEMENT OF THE IMMOBILE PATIENT WITH MS

Patients with MS may become immobile either due to disease progression causing handicap, or during periods of relapse. Whether patients become wheelchair or bed-bound, correct physical management remains essential to their well-being.

Respiratory inadequacy must be prevented so as to avert chest infections, partial lung collapse, accumulation of sputum and cyanosis. A correct breathing pattern should be established by teaching deep breathing exercises in recumbent and/or sitting positions, and checks made to ensure air entry to all areas of the lungs.

Circulatory stasis, particularly of the lower limbs, must be avoided as this increases the risk of deep vein thrombosis. Active exercises of rhythmic contraction and relaxation will employ a muscle pump mechanism to aid venous return. If no active muscle contraction is possible, passive manipulation and massage may be required, or a mechanical aid employed.

Spastic and fixed contractures can be prevented by moving joints through full passive ranges of movement. Correct posture and positioning to ensure prolonged stretch of muscle groups affected by hypertonia should become habitual, and daily prone lying is essential for the immobile patient.

Pressure area care to prevent the development of pressure sores is a vital part of the management programme. Correct support and positioning of the body and limbs to avoid pressure points is essential, and regular turning or change in position is necessary day and night. In addition, successful prevention of respiratory and circulatory stasis, contractures and deformities will also help the prevention of pressure sores.

Successful management of the immobile patient relies on all preventative and maintenance regimens being incorporated into daily life. The physiotherapists will need to assume an educative and supervisory role and pass on basic handling and treatment skills to all carers, both lay and professional. In addition, safe and efficient ways of turning, lifting and transferring the immobile patient should be shown. Follow-up by the physiotherapist is essential to ensure that instructions are being correctly executed, to change those instructions if the circumstances of the patient or carers have changed, and to give support and reassurance to carers.

The physical management of MS, therefore, although initiated and directed by the physiotherapist, is not exclusive to therapy sessions alone. The patient and family should be made aware of what constitutes good movement, and encouraged by the physiotherapist to achieve it rather than to develop poor habits of movement. The physiotherapist and patient should therefore work together in partnership so that the benefits of therapy are translated into activities used for everyday life.

REFERENCES

Ashburn, A. and De Souza, L.H. (1988) An approach to the management of multiple sclerosis. *Physiotherapy Practice*, 4, 139–45.

Bach-y-Rita, P. (1980) Brain plasticity as a basis for therapeutic procedure, in *Recovery of Function: Theoretical Considerations for Brain Injury Rehabilitation* (ed. P. Bach-y-Rita) Hans Huber Publishers, Stuttgart, Vienna.

Bobath, B. (1978) *Adult Hemiplegia: Evaluation and Treatment*, 2nd edn. Heinemann, London.

Bouillaud (1846) Referred to by R. Garcin, in *Handbook of Neurology* (eds P.J. Vinken and G.W. Bruyn) Vol.1. Amsterdam, North Holland Publishing Co. 1975, pp. 309–55.

Carr, J.H. and Shepherd, R.B. (1987) *A Motor Re-learning Programme for Stroke*, 2nd edn. Heinemann, London.

De Souza, L.H. (1983) The effects of sensation and motivation on regaining movement control following stroke. *Physiotherapy*, **60**, 238–40.

De Souza, L.H. (1984) A different approach to physiotherapy for multiple sclerosis patients. *Physiotherapy*, **70**, 429–32.

De Souza, L.H. and Musa, I. (1987) The measurement and assessment of spasticity. *Clinical Rehabilitation*, **1**, 89–96.

Frenkel, H.S. (1890) Die Therapie atactisher Bewegunstorugen. *Munchen Medizin Weschrift*, **37**, 917.

Gardiner, M.D. (1976) *The Principles of Exercise Therapy*. G. Bell and Sons, London.

Globus, A., Rosenzweig, M.R., Bennett, E.L. *et al.* (1973) Effects of differential experience on dendritic spine counts. *Journal of Comparative Physiology and Psychology*, **82**, 175–81.

Goff, B. (1976) Grading of spasticity and its effect on voluntary movement. *Physiotherapy*, **62**, 358–61.

Greenough, W.T. (1976) Enduring brain effects of differential experience in training, in *Neural Mechanisms of Learning and Memory* (eds M.R. Rosenzweig and E.L. Bennett). MIT Press, Cambridge, Massachusetts, pp. 255–78.

Hewer, R.L. (1980) Multiple sclerosis management and rehabilitation. *International Rehabilitation Medicine*, **2**, 116–25.

Jones, B. (1974) The importance of memory traces of motor efferent discharges for learning skilled movements. *Developmental Medicine and Child Neurology*, **16**, 620–8.

Knott, M. and Voss, D.E. (1968) *Proprioceptive Neuromuscular Facilitation*, 2nd edn. Harper and Row, New York.

Mazzuca, S.A. (1982) Does patient education in chronic disease have therapeutic values? *Journal of Chronic Disease*, **35**, 521–9.

Mead, S. and Knott, M. (1960) A six year evaluation of PNF techniques. *Proceedings of the 3rd International Congress of Physical Medicine*, Chicago, 1960.

Morgan, M.H. (1980) Ataxia – its causes, measurement and management. *International Rehabilitation Medicine*, **2**, 126–32.

Morgan, M.H., Hewer, R.L. and Cooper, R. (1975) Application of an objective method of assessing intention tremor – a further study on the use of weights to reduce intention tremor. *Journal of Neurology, Neurosurgery and Psychiatry,* **38**, 259–64.

Odeen, I. (1981) Reduction of muscular hypertonus by long-term muscle stretch. *Scandinavian Journal of Rehabilitation Medicine,* **13**, 93–9.

Raisman, G. and Field, P.M. (1973) A quantitative investigation of the development of collateral re-innervation of the septal nuclei. *Brain Research,* **50**, 241–64.

Roberts, T.D.M. (1978) *Neurophysiology of Postural Mechanisms,* 2nd edn. Butterworths, London.

Todd, J. (1982) Physiotherapy and multiple sclerosis, in *Progress in Multiple Sclerosis* (eds R. Capildeo and A. Maxwell). Macmillan Press, Hong Kong, pp. 31–44.

Wall, P.D. (1980) Mechanisms of plasticity of connection following damage in adult mammalian nervous system. in *Recovery of function: theoretical considerations for brain injury rehabilitation* (ed. P. Bach-y-Rita). Hans Huber, Bern, Stuttgart, Vienna, pp. 91–105.

5

Occupational therapy

Lorraine H. De Souza

In general, the occupational therapist (OT) will be called upon to help people with multiple sclerosis (MS) to achieve the best level of independent living as possible. The majority of MS cases generally referred are people with a permanent, and often severe, disability or handicap. Before this stage of disability is reached there are several areas of care and management where occupational therapy has much to offer. Unfortunately, however, when earlier referrals to OTs do not take place, opportunities for patients to utilize a valuable resource are wasted, and hence therapists generally see MS patients only when they are incapacitated by the disease. Yet before stages of severe disability are reached, many MS patients experience disorders of functioning which limit their capabilities for independent living. Appropriate occupational therapy, aimed at increasing functional ability, can help to extend the capacity for independent living, and open up opportunities for people with MS to make choices about the lives they wish to live.

This chapter will discuss areas of management where OTs may be used to good effect in helping people and families live with MS.

RECOVERY FROM RELAPSES

Many first encounters between OTs and people with MS take place in hospital when patients have suffered an exacerbation of the disease. A relapse which is severe enough to warrant hospitalization of the MS patient may have caused fairly extensive incapacitation. Some of the apparent disability will be temporary, and although a degree of recovery generally occurs, no-one can predict how much. The OT will need to work with the patient in order to develop strategies for self-care. The main aim of treatment is to re-establish activities of independent daily living at levels as close as possible to those experienced by the MS patient before the relapse. Activities such as washing, dressing, grooming, toileting and eating require first assessment, and then therapeutic intervention at the earliest opportunities. As recovery occurs, or the patient's condition becomes more stable, other activities such as transferring should be encouraged. Signs of a continuing recovery from relapse indicate changing treatment strategies so that a progression towards more independence in daily living activities is planned for as therapy continues.

A regular re-evaluation for necessary and appropriate aids for daily living is required, with appliances being given with instructions in their use and exchanged for others as recovery progresses. It is important that patients are encouraged and supported by the OT to strive for independence in self-care activities even in the early stages after a relapse. However, attention should be taken to the levels of fatigue experienced by the patient when attempting different tasks and accounted for in the therapy programme.

In the later stages of the therapy programme assessment followed by advice and treatment for home-making skills, work and leisure activities will be required. Towards the end of the period a comparison between the patient's pre-relapse level of independence and current status by the OT will indicate the extent to which the damage to the central nervous system caused by the disease has resulted in functional impairment. A record of the final assessment and its comparisons with the patient's pre-relapse level of independence forms the basis of a discharge report which should then be passed on to the community care team.

Shortly before, or soon after, the MS patient returns home from hospital a home visit by the OT will be required.

HOME VISITING

The main purposes for the OT to carry out a home visit are firstly to observe and assess the MS patient's abilities in daily living activities, secondly to identify areas of difficulties or problems with activities, and thirdly to determine whether or not aids and structural adaptations to the home are necessary for activities. The main advantage of seeing patients in their own homes is that abilities in daily living activities can be judged within the context of the environment in which they must be carried out.

The home environment consists of several inter-dependent aspects, all of which the therapist will need to identify and gauge in order to help the patient exploit all his capabilities.

The type of house, the location of various rooms, positions of stairs or steps with existing bannisters and rails will all require noting. The OT should also notice the positions of major pieces of furniture, and the locations of the focal points in each room. Access to the home and accessibility between the various rooms are also important.

Home environment is also provided by the patient's family and the OT needs to be observant and sensitive of the family dynamics. It is important to note, without appearing to be inquisitive, the following:

1. What is the family role of the MS patient, e.g. father, mother, child?
2. Does the family appear supportive towards the relative with MS?
3. How many people live in the family home?
4. Who are the dependent relatives? e.g. child, elderly person.
5. Who are the primary carers and providers?
6. Who is at home during the day, and when?
7. Is there an extended family living in the area?

During a home visit, therefore, the OT is in a position to assess the ability of the MS patient to reassume his individual patterns of daily living in the context of family life.

EVALUATING ACTIVITIES OF DAILY LIVING

Activities of daily living (ADL) include the personal care activities, which most patients aspire to being totally independent with, and more general activities relevant to their social lives (Benjamin, 1976). Assessment of ADL, and reassessment at regular intervals, provides a record of the levels of ability and independence of each individual MS patient. These levels may fluctuate, for example during periods of relapse and recovery, or change due to disease progression or in response to therapeutic programmes.

There are numerous forms available for evaluating ADL, and the one chosen must depend on the OT's requirement. Two types of method available as tools for the OT are the ADL assessment and the ADL index. Nichols (1976) describes the ADL assessment as being suitable to use as a record of a patient's accomplishments and future potential, and provides information relevant for day-to-day planning and adjustment of treatment programmes. The ADL index is more suited to providing ordered records of the patient's abilities and can be used for assessing, monitoring change and screening patients.

The various advantages and disadvantages of ADL assessments, indices and scales have been critically reviewed by Ashburn (1986) and Eakin (1989). It is pointed out that the interpretation of the ADL information is as important as the information itself. A major fault of many ADL indices is their failure to record small functional changes due to their insensitivity. For the same reason many may produce a ceiling effect implying that the patient has stopped making progress when this may not be the case (Ashburn, 1986).

One parameter rarely recorded with ADL is the time taken by patients to complete tasks. Activities which can be completed by the patient, but are too time consuming, may not be attempted at home. The OT should be aware of the amount of time taken by each patient to carry out various ADL activities and provide advice and strategies to help when tasks take abnormally long to complete. The time factor has important implications if the patient suffers from fatigue, and if time-consuming tasks disrupt the family routine. If the patient is able to complete ADL tasks progressively quicker and therefore use energy more efficiently, progress is being made. By using time as an additional feature of ADL evaluation the OT may communicate this progress to the patient, and provide further encouragement.

HELPING PATIENTS PLAN DAILY LIVING

The activities involved in day-to-day living are invariably not all recorded by ADL assessments and indices. Some activities, such as eating and dressing, are common to all people, but others such as driving or going to work may only be relevant to some. The life styles of people are often more restricted in choice and aspirations when MS must also be taken into account.

The OT, out of all the professional carers, is the person with the necessary relevant skills who can help the MS patient and the family plan daily living for the life style they wish to lead.

As part of assessment, the OT needs to determine the limitations to activities caused by the MS itself. The effects of physical disability, fatigue and poor memory all have major impact on normal daily living. Patients are faced with choices, often unwelcome ones, imposed by the MS, and like everyone else may make good or bad decisions. A bad decision by the MS patient who may be physically, psychologically or emotionally vulnerable, could have a profound effect on personal well-being and that of the family unit.

The OT can help patients to make the correct choices for themselves by working with them to produce a well thought-out plan of daily living. In doing this, the therapist must beware of dictating to the patient what ought to be done, and how it should be done. She should also be careful not to present a negative attitude by reminding the patient too often of what is beyond his capabilities. On the other hand, the therapist must alert the patient to unsafe practices, and the possible negative consequences of some of the choices he wishes to make. In addition, the OT should be prepared for the occasions when the patient will not take his/her advice and he/she should resist showing disapproval or placing blame. The therapist should also be wary of consciously or subconsciously judging the patient's way of living, and success at tasks, by her own standards. A successful therapist–patient relationship is essential in order to work in a manner where the OT's professional expertise can be accessed and utilized by the patient when developing a plan for daily living.

DEVELOPING A DAILY LIVING PLAN

To begin with, the OT should inform the patient about how he has performed on the ADL evaluation. They will need to discuss the various activities relevant to an average day. The therapist should encourage the patient to identify the tasks required by the average day, and to decide which are the most essential activities.

Essential activities are those which must be performed for personal reasons, such as going to the toilet or eating a meal, or for family reasons such as taking or fetching children from school. Some essential tasks may be able to be shifted around in time during the day, while others may have to be carried out at a specific time of day. Other daily activities can be organized around those which are essential, and the effects of the symptoms of MS accounted for in the plan.

The daily pattern of fatigue should be first determined by the OT. Activities requiring the most energy or concentration should be programmed at times of the day when the patient feels least fatigued. The use of rest periods or a short mid-day sleep can be counselled in order to alleviate fatigue so that necessary tasks can be carried out in the late afternoon or evening. Fetching children from school, caring for them by, for example, providing their meals, helping with schoolwork and preparing them for bed, may be seen as priority tasks for mothers who have MS. Yet it is the late afternoon and evening when they may feel most fatigued. The OT can help mothers to plan the day's activities and to use rest periods in order to ensure that they have a good chance of saving enough energy during the day to be able to interact with their children when they return home from school.

CAPABILITY AND PERFORMANCE

It has been noted that patients often do not perform all the activities of daily living that they are capable of carrying out (Nichols, 1976). Staples and Lincoln (1979) discovered discrepancies between MS patients' ability to perform ADL as assessed by OTs in a rehabilitation unit, and the activities which were carried out by patients and reported by their relatives. Such discrepancies are not exclusive to MS, but have also been reported for stroke patients (Andrews and Stewart, 1979). These results however may not be specific to the diagnostic groups studied, but may be a more general feature of behaviour (Lincoln, 1981).

Most people do not carry out all the daily living tasks that they are capable of. Some tasks may be delegated to other family members for the sake of convenience, while household tasks may be purposely given to an employed home help in order to release leisure time. Again, other tasks, such as washing up the dishes, may be given to children as part of their upbringing discipline. Within a family unit there is often a division of labour so that various activities required to keep the household running smoothly are shared out among the members.

There may be other, more subtle reasons why MS patients do not perform all the activities that they are capable of carrying out. Activities may be too laborious and fatiguing, or may not be carried out to the individual's standards of cleanliness or hygiene, and are not attempted at all (De Souza, 1984). Some MS patients, perhaps insecure in their relationships, may deliberately behave in a more helpless manner in order to gain more physical and intimate contact with their partners.

When patients with MS do not perform all the ADL which they

are capable of, reasons should be sought by the OT. Some reasons are quite valid within the context of an individual's family and social life and, therefore, it cannot be presumed that non-performance of tasks is due to the MS.

Where MS is the cause of the patient being unable to carry out tasks he wants to do, the OT can help with positive interventions. The appropriate occupational therapy, advice, aids or appliances may enable the MS patient to perform the desired activities. If the OT suspects that over-dependency on the carer is due to psychological or emotional reasons, then referral to a counsellor may be appropriate.

AIDS FOR INDEPENDENT LIVING

For many MS patients who become disabled due to disease progression the utilization of aids may be the sole means of retaining independence in ADL. A comprehensive assessment by the OT is necessary to indicate which types of aids may be useful to the patient. Attention should be given to the following areas where deficits could influence the type of aid suggested:

1. Manual dexterity;
2. physical capacity;
3. sensory function;
4. visual discrimination;
5. short-term and long-term memory.

Although aids will be given to compensate for some physical deficits, certain physical abilities will be required so that they may be successfully used. The OT's judgement comes into play, as it is important that the MS patient does not fail to use the aid successfully. Such a failure may result in the patient rejecting the aid, feeling demoralized, and being suspicious of aids which may be introduced in the future.

The patient should be encouraged by the OT to participate in the decisions about aids, and, if possible, be allowed to choose an aid from a range which is appropriate and available. The use of an aid should not be forced upon the patient no matter how necessary its use may appear. Patience and persuasion are often required for those with MS who view the necessity for an aid as a sign that the disease has made them worse.

With many MS patients the giving of an aid is only the start of the OT's work. Some will require only a simple explanation and a single demonstration to use the aid successfully. Others may require more intense instructions. Those with poor vision may need to be shown several times how to use an aid, and perhaps, also, a great deal of verbal instructions and trials under supervision. Likewise, patients who have memory dysfunction due to MS may need to be shown several times how to use aids by the OT. It is often useful to give clearly written instructions, with pictures or diagrams if possible, with the aid as a source of reference for the MS patient. Such instructions may be given as a matter of course with aids as often patients are unaware of early signs of memory loss, or believe that their visual loss is less than it really is, and even a comprehensive OT assessment may not reveal the full extent of these deficits.

In a long-term plan of management it will be necessary to review the aids used by each individual at regular intervals. As the disease progresses, some aids may become redundant and should be exchanged for others which are more appropriate. A regular review can also identify aids which have broken or become worn out from use. All non-functioning aids should be withdrawn as they may be hazards to safety if patients persist in using them, or be considered as 'useless' or 'unreliable' and not be used at all.

HOME ADAPTATIONS

Most patients disabled by MS will require some adaptations to their home. These may range from a simple, strategically placed grab-rail, to complete re-fitting of rooms for wheelchair use. The OT may be asked to provide assessments and reports for the health care team and the GP, and be expected to liaise with those concerned in making the home adaptations, such as architects, electricians and builders. His/her professional experience and recommendations will be sought as decisions are made about adapting a patient's home for living with a disability.

All adaptations to the house will have advantages and disadvantages, not all of which may be obvious. Discussions with the patient and family will reveal the pros and cons of each adaptation from each person's point of view. As many structural adaptations are both expensive, and largely irreversible, the OT should be convinced that it is not only necessary, but also wanted by the MS patient and family.

It should be remembered that houses are not just buildings of bricks and mortar, but also have emotional, psychological and social value to the inhabitants. This is even more the case when the house is also home to a family. The OT should strive for a family decision on all proposed adaptations, and remember that the house is not just space to live in, but also the environment in which people with MS and their families receive visitors, maintain many different types of relationships and raise their children. Consultation is therefore essential, and care should be taken to allow as much choice as possible in terms of style, design and colour schemes.

In our present society, houses are also the one major financial investment for those who are able to be home owners. While some adaptations, such as an extra downstairs toilet, may add to the value of the house, others such as bathroom hoists may detract from its value. Obvious and severe structural changes may make the house difficult to sell if the family wants to, or has to, move.

When advising on home adaptations, the OT will need to take into consideration all those various factors. The best advice and help the OT can give may be to provide the necessary knowledge and information to allow the MS patient and family to reach their own decisions.

WORK

The majority of people who have MS are in young adulthood, and therefore would expect to be part of the workforce, and be able to pursue careers. Occupational therapists have a role in helping MS patients to explore their vocational capabilities and interests.

Functionally the disabilities can be viewed in two major categories: first, the lack of work skills, habits and behaviour, and secondly neurophysiological impairments. The OT can provide the patient with a progressive series of learning experiences which will facilitate appropriate vocational decisions, and develop work habits which are necessary for the chosen employment (Ad Hoc Committee, 1980). In order to implement therapy for vocational rehabilitation, the OT will need to evaluate each individual. Many factors need to be taken into account. What are the patient's interests and aspirations? Does the patient have a realistic goal in mind? What is the extent of the patient's job experience and what type of work is available in the local community? Some of these answers may be obtained by the OT working in conjunction with the Disablement

Resettlement Officer (DRO), local employment agencies or job centres.

The OT evaluates by applying practical and reality-based assessment techniques. The objectives, as stated by the American Occupational Therapy Association's policy document (1980), are the following:

1. Testing and evaluating work abilities related to specific job tasks;
2. assessing the patient's learning ability and retention of skills;
3. evaluation of the physical, psychological, and social factors such as work tolerance, habits, and inter-personal qualities.

The applications of work evaluation and assessments have been described by Matheson (1982) and Matheson and Ogden (1983).

Part of OT work with MS patients may include careful counselling to help make career choices where MS will have less impact. Some patients may be encouraged to consider steering their careers in a slightly different direction than was first envisaged. The OT can help with advice about vocational training and education, and about the different aids and adaptations that can make various job tasks easier.

Any contact with a patient's place of work must only be made with permission. Many with MS do not tell their work colleagues or managers of the condition in case it prejudices their chances of promotion, or puts their job at risk.

The role of the OT in the fairly new area of work-related programmes and assessments is extensively described by Jacobs (1985).

LEISURE

There has been a tendency for OTs to move away from the use of expressive and creative activities as part of treatment. Some may feel that these are out-dated treatment modes, while others that they give a false impression of the nature of occupational therapy.

The prejudices of individual therapists, however, should not override the needs of their patients. The introduction of a new craft or interest may bring much pleasure as well as improvement in function for some patients. For many with MS, facing progressively more leisure time as their disease advances, the benefits of learning new activities should not be underestimated. Art and handicrafts as a

63

therapeutic medium also teach skill, dexterity, precision and ingenuity, while at the same time providing an outlet for emotional and creative qualities in patients.

For some patients, mostly women, the ability to sew, embroider, mend, darn and knit may constitute their major practical contribution to the family. Part of the OT's work is to determine what each individual patient can do and would like to do. Although, as with other activities, craftwork should not be imposed on patients, those who have an urge to pursue such activities need to be encouraged and helped by the therapists involved.

Music, drama, or creative writing may likewise provide modes of expression for individual patients. Some may have a natural talent for such activities and should be encouraged. For some patients the ability to use and express their creative talents is valuable, emotionally and psychologically, as it emphasizes their individuality and provides a medium for interaction with like-minded people in the world at large.

There are many outdoor pursuits and sports which are suitable and available for people with disabilities (Croucher, 1981). Many involve joining a group or club, which has the added advantage of increasing opportunities for social contact. Advice can be offered about local availability of sports activities. It is also important to offer help to MS patients wishing to include sport in their life styles. Strategies to cope with fatigue and poor concentration may be provided by OTs in order to help patients enjoy their sport with minimum adverse effects. Some sports activities, such as swimming (Gehlsen, Grigsby and Winant, 1984; Trussell, 1971) and horse riding (Saywell, 1975) may also provide suitable therapeutic media for treatment.

Not all outdoor activities demand physical ability or a great deal of exertion and some, for example angling (Warren, 1988), can provide enjoyment and relaxation for even severely disabled people. Many people with MS may prefer participation as a spectator, and information can be provided concerning accessibility to venues (RADAR, 1980).

MOTHERHOOD

Nearly all surveys of MS agree that women are more likely than men to have the disease. Acheson (1977), for example, concluded that women were 40% more at risk from the disease than men, while Kurtzke, Beebe and Norman (1979) quote the risk at 80% greater.

In addition, there is general agreement that the mean age of onset is between 29 and 30 years (Matthews *et al.,* 1985; p.49). The epidemiological data provides evidence that large numbers of women experience the onset of MS in the middle of their child-bearing years.

Although, in the past, it was thought that pregnancy had an adverse effect on progression of MS, more recent opinion is that this is not the case (see Chapter 11). Women with MS who wish to have a child may have many anxieties related to the disease. The OT is in a position to help to alleviate some of these anxieties by offering counselling, support and practical aid.

Many health workers who become involved with women during anti-natal and post-natal care may know very little about MS or, more specifically, about MS as experienced by the individual. Using knowledge from assessment and intervention, the OT can act as a source of information for the other health care professionals. For example, fatigue is often experienced by both MS people and pregnant women, but the OT, from experience of an individual, can identify how much may be due to the MS and how much may be additional and due to the pregnancy.

Several physical changes experienced in pregnancy are also experienced by women with MS, and an easy option may be to blame the MS. Examples of such symptoms are urinary incontinence, swollen limbs and water retention, and a range of unusual sensory disturbances. Where doubt exists, patients should always be advised to consult their doctor. The OT, however, can do much to reassure the pregnant patient, when physical changes are due to the pregnancy, that they are not due to the MS progressing.

The event of pregnancy for women who have disabilities may raise anxieties about their ability to cope, physically and mentally, with a newborn infant and with raising the child. Such anxieties may be expressed by both patients and professionals (National Childbirth Trust, 1984). The professional however should take care not to give opinion and advice based upon personal views of disabled mothers. Women with MS and their partners may have to confront many issues in the light of the disease and an uncertain future. Some of these issues are raised by Robinson (1988; pp. 68–73), and information for MS patients about pregnancy and having a baby is available (Forti and Segal, 1987).

Some mothers with MS who have symptoms affecting their physical abilities will benefit from intervention of an OT. Practical help and advice can encourage the mother to adapt her life style in an appropriate manner to manage best both the new baby and the MS. Re-assessment of fatigue patterns and ADL are called for, as the nature of both will be radically changed when the new baby arrives. On the basis of assessment, appropriate management strategies, aids or adaptations can be decided.

One example of a management strategy for fatigue in a breast-feeding mother may be to indicate positions where it is possible to feed the infant and rest at the same time, for example a side-lying position, where with careful placement of pillows the mother's arms do not become fatigued from holding the infant for feeding. This and other lying positions may be useful when mothers are breast-feeding new babies through the night.

In the day-time, a simple aid, like a sling across the mother's chest, can also help to alleviate tiredness in the arms. In this way the mother can keep her baby close to her without needing constantly to hold it in her arms, and this may be a useful aid to breast-feeding mothers.

The OT may need to teach the mother with MS the movement skills required to change nappies, wash and bath her baby. In some cases adaptations will need to be considered so that the mother can carry out baby-care tasks from a wheelchair, or in a sitting position if she cannot stand for any period of time. The acquisition of movement skills will also encourage confidence in the mother when handling her baby, and enhance enjoyment and satisfaction for her in her new role as a mother.

The OT can aid the facilitation of mother–child interactions, not only through improving the MS mother's handling skills, but also by encouraging her to play with her child. Postures and positions which will put mother and child in situations where easy physical and eye contact are possible should be advised and explored. In some cases play activities may need to be suggested and developed.

In all interventions with the MS mother, the OT should be capable of assuming a supportive role. This includes supporting the mother in her decisions about how she wishes to parent, and helping her to communicate and discuss her choices with others who are involved.

The above is also applicable, though in slightly different manner, when it is the father who has MS. The development of parenting skills is as important for the father in helping him assume his new role. Whichever parent has MS, the OT is in a position to help and advise, and by doing so in a sensitive and professional manner can prevent the parent with MS from becoming unnecessarily isolated, or distanced from the child.

Finally, not all mothers, whether or not they have MS, do everything all the time for their babies. The supportive work of the OT includes reassuring the patient that she is a 'good mother', and helping to rationalize any fears she may have about being a 'bad mother'. Sometimes it is helpful to remind patients that, with parenthood, 'being' is more important than 'doing'.

THE SEVERELY DISABLED MS PATIENT

A small percentage of those with MS will experience disease progression to a state where they are severely disabled (Scheinberg *et al.*, 1984). For many, the ability to lead an independent life will be significantly compromised, and they may come to depend partially or totally on others.

The emphasis of occupational therapy for severely disabled MS patients should be to maintain residual abilities for as long as is possible, and to prevent the development of complications. The diligent and regular use of assessment will help to identify the patient's residual abilities, and give early warning of any complications arising.

As the MS patient becomes progressively more incapacitated, the focus of OT shifts slightly. The abilities and needs of carers must now be encompassed much more than before in a plan of management. The OT is in a position to maintain a watching brief on the carers, to identify when and where the burden of care becomes unbearable for them, and to initiate the necessary support services well in advance of crisis situations. The needs of carers in these situations cannot be underestimated (Oliver, 1985). Where the MS patient is permanently dependent on others for day-to-day care the OT can provide support, teach transferring techniques and provide aids for the benefit of carers.

Transferring

All patients, even the most severely incapacitated, will require transferring during the day. The OT should instruct the carer in safe, efficient and effective ways of transferring the MS patient. Some carers are able and prefer to carry out transfers by physical effort alone, others may welcome the use of hoists (Tarling, 1980) or transfer boards. In all transfers any co-operation, however small, from the MS patient should be encouraged.

Some transfers may be beyond the ability of a single carer, and two people may need to be instructed and taught how to work as a team when lifting the patient. In some cases district nursing or care attendant services may need to be brought in to help with, for example, bathing.

All people involved in transferring the patient should be made aware of the danger of causing tears or abrasions to the skin of the buttocks. This should be avoided at all costs as skin breakdown or infection can easily lead to pressure sores.

Pressure area care

The OT can provide carers with several strategies for positioning and changing the posture of the MS patient. Attention should be drawn to the benefits of a good sitting posture in chairs and wheelchairs (Pope, 1985a,b). Modification of cushions may be considered in order to reduce pressure on weight-bearing points (Krouskop and Garber, 1984). Some simple bed and chair coverings, such as sheepskins, may help, and some patients may require extra protection, such as heel cradles, for particularly vulnerable areas.

Continence

There is probably nothing as distressing and humiliating as being wet from incontinence. Apart from this, such a situation is undesirable as the acidity of urine has a detrimental effect on the skin. For many with MS, the 'toilet transfer' is extremely difficult, and the OT will need to assess this activity *in situ*, to determine the best movement strategies and most appropriate aids and adaptations for each individual. Nocturia is a common symptom in MS, and the provision of a commode in the bedroom for night use may be necessary. Where a commode is supplied, provision should also be made for its emptying, cleansing and sanitizing.

The majority of MS patients experiencing incontinence will also benefit from referral to continence advisors.

The OT can also help women with MS to manage menstrual hygiene (Duckworth, 1986).

Feeding

For many with MS the ability to eat and drink, at least partly by their own ability, is the last bastion of independent living. There are a multitude of feeding aids available for the disabled, and the OT's knowledge and skill should ensure that the most appropriate ones are provided. Some foods are easier to eat than others, and discussion with a dietitian can help the OT to suggest those which are both easy to eat and nutritionally valuable. Patients who have chewing and swallowing dysfunction should be referred to the speech therapist for assessment and advice (see Chapter 6).

Environmental control

With the advent of new technology, there are now available many electronic systems which will control household equipment. With these systems some severely disabled people may be able to achieve a degree of independence. Often a specialist assessment is required to find the correct system for an individual, and all patients will need teaching and practice in order to use them to best effect. The use of technology as tools for living has been discussed by Bray and Wright (1980).

SUMMARY

The diversity of disabilities in MS challenges the capabilities of occupational therapists. Yet OTs are in the unique position to utilize the many treatment media available to them in order to treat the whole person. Ideally, the 'occupation' on which the 'therapy' is based is initiated by the MS patient, and nurtured by the OT via therapeutic interventions. This type of partnership provides the means and opportunities necessary to enable the MS patient to lead the life he or she chooses to live.

REFERENCES

Acheson, E.D. (1977) Epidemiology of multiple sclerosis. *British Medical Bulletin,* **33**, 9–14.
Ad Hoc Committee of the Commission on Practice (1980) The role of

occupational therapy in the vocational rehabilitation process: official position paper. *American Journal of Occupational Therapy,* **34**, 881.

Andrews, K. and Stewart, J. (1979) Stroke recovery: he can but does he? *Rheumatology and Rehabilitation,* **18**, 43–8.

Ashburn, A. (1986) Methods of assessing the physical disabilities of stroke patients. *Physiotherapy Practice,* **2**, 59–62.

Benjamin, J. (1976) The Northwick Park A.D.L. Index. *Occupational Therapy,* **39**, 301–6.

Bray, J. and Wright, S. (eds) (1980) *The Use of Technology in the Care of the Elderly and the Disabled: Tools for living.* Francis Pinter Ltd., London.

Croucher, N. (1981) *Outdoor Pursuits for Disabled People.* Disabled Living Foundation, London.

De Souza, L.H. (1984) A different approach to physiotherapy for multiple sclerosis patients. *Physiotherapy,* **70**(11), 429–32.

Duckworth, B. (1986) Overview of menstrual management for disabled women. *Canadian Journal of Occupational Therapy,* **53**(1), 25–9.

Eakin, P. (1989) Assessments of activities of daily living: a critical review. *British Journal of Occupational Therapy,* **52**(1), 11–15.

Forti, A.D. and Segal, J. (1987) *MS and Pregnancy.* ARMS (Action and Research for Multiple Sclerosis) Publication, Stansted, Essex.

Gehlsen, G.M., Grigsby, S.A. and Winant, D.M. (1984) Effects of an aquatic fitness program on the muscular strength and endurance of patients with multiple sclerosis. *Physical Therapy,* **64**(5), 653–7.

Jacobs, K. (1985) *Occupational Therapy: Work-related programs and assessments.* Little, Brown and Co., Boston and Toronto.

Krouskop, T.A. and Garber, S.L. (1984) Wheelchair cushion modification and its effects on pressure. *Archives of Physical Medicine and Rehabilitation,* **65**, 579–83.

Kurtzke, J.F., Beebe, G.W. and Norman, J.E. (1979) Epidemiology of multiple sclerosis in U.S. veterans 1: Race, sex, and geographic distribution. *Neurology,* **29**, 1228–35.

Lincoln, N.B. (1981) Discrepancies between capabilities and performance of activities of daily living in multiple sclerosis. *International Rehabilitation Medicine,* **3**, 84–8.

Matheson, L.N. (1982) *Work Capacity Evaluation: A training manual for occupational therapists.* Rehab. Inst. of Southern California, Trabuco Canyon, California.

Matheson, L.N. and Ogden, L.D. (1983) *Work Tolerance Screening.* Rehab.Inst.of Southern California, Trabuco Canyon, California.

Matthews, W.B., Acheson, E.D., Batchelor, J.R. *et al.* (eds) (1985) *McAlpine's Multiple Sclerosis.* Churchill Livingstone, London.

National Childbirth Trust (1984) *The Emotions and Experiences of Disabled Mothers.* National Childbirth Trust, London.

Nichols, P. (1976) Are ADL indices of any value? *Occupational Therapy,* **39**(6), 160–3.

Oliver, M. (1985) Who cares for the carers? *Self Health* No.8.

Pope, P. (1985a) A study of instability in relation to posture in the wheelchair. *Physiotherapy,* **71**, 124–9.

Pope, P. (1985b) Proposals for the improvement of the unstable postural condition and some cautionary notes. *Physiotherapy*, **71**, 129–31.

Robinson, I. (1988) *Multiple Sclerosis*. Routledge, London.

Royal Association for Disability and Rehabilitation (RADAR) (1980) *Sports and Leisure Access Guide for the Disabled Spectator*. RADAR, London.

Saywell, S.Y. (1975) Riding and ataxia. *Physiotherapy*, **61**(11), 334–5.

Scheinberg, L., Kalb, R., Larocca, N. *et al.* (1984) The doctor–patient relationship in multiple sclerosis, in *The Diagnosis of Multiple Sclerosis* (ed. C.M. Poser) Thieme-Stratton Inc., New York, pp. 205–15.

Staples, D. and Lincoln, N.B. (1979) Intellectual impairment in multiple sclerosis and its relation to functional abilities. *Rheumatology and Rehabilitation*, **18**, 153–60.

Tarling, C. (1980) *Hoists and their Use*. Heinemann Medical Books, London.

Trussell, E.C. (1971) Swimming for the disabled. *Physiotherapy*, **57**(10), 461–6.

Warren, L.D. (1988) The Handicapped Anglers Trust. *Clinical Rehabilitation*, **2**, 161–2.

6

Communication disorders

Pamela Enderby

The communication disorders associated with multiple sclerosis can be more complex in nature and presentation than has been generally accepted. Usually, textbooks and articles have focused on the incidence and presentation of dysarthria; rarely have dysphasia, hearing loss, elective mutism or dysphonia been mentioned, and yet they are certainly known to be features of the various communication problems which may present in the course of the disease.

DYSARTHRIA

Charcot (1877) placed dysarthria in the triad of symptoms along with nystagmus and intention tremor and suggested these were the identifying characteristics of MS. He did not use the term dysarthria but referred to 'scanning speech', that is prolonged phonation of words with slow and slurred articulation. Ivers and Goldstein (1963) have demonstrated that dysarthria is not a universal characteristic of MS. They found 19% with this speech impairment and that it was a presenting symptom in only 2% of their sample. Kurtzke (1983) suggested a similar prevalence figure for dysarthria in MS (20%) which is different to the Mayo Clinic study which suggested a figure of 41% (Darley, Brown and Goldstein, 1972). The later study, whose main investigator was a speech therapist, had different inclusion criteria from the former studies conducted by neurologists. Whereas a speech therapist would identify hypernasality related to neuromotor velopharyngeal insufficiency as dysarthria, others may not, as the defect would mostly alter the quality of speech rather than intelligibility.

A study using a self-reporting technique in a postal survey of 656 individuals with MS found that 23% reported a 'speech and/or communication disorder' (Beukelman, Kraft and Freal, 1985). Thus the prevalence of dysarthria can be said to be between 19% and 41% depending on the interpretation of what dysarthria is and the methods used.

Nature of the dysarthria

Charcot (1877) described the speech of persons with MS as being slow and drawling, sometimes unintelligible, and the words spoken as 'measured and scanned' with a pause between syllables which are pronounced slowly and hesitantly. He noted that the dysarthria may hardly be perceptible at onset by may become incomprehensible, and at times 'it becomes suddenly aggravated, as if in paroxysms, and then grows temporarily better'. This description tallies with that associated with cerebellar disturbance and has been cited in many subsequent medical textbooks.

Not all patients with dysarthria will have the cerebellar type; it is to be expected that the underlying neurological lesions would affect the nature of the neuromotor speech disorder. Darley, Aronson and Brown (1975) grouped the MS patients in their study into eight neurologic groups: spinal, cerebral, brainstem cerebellar, cerebral plus brainstem, brainstem plus cerebellar, cerebral plus cerebellar and cerebral, brainstem and cerebellar.

The groups shared some speech abnormalities. The most frequent deviations were impaired loudness control (77%) and harsh voice quality (72%). About half the subjects had defective articulation (46%). Impaired emphasis was noted in 39%, which related to prosodic characteristics including the patient's rate of speech, phrasing, vocal pitch and volume variations. Approximately a quarter (24%) had some degree of hypernasality, inappropriate pitch level (24%) and breathiness (22%). The latter probably related to decreased vital capacity (35%).

The study concluded that there were features of speech that differed according to the neurological impairment, and that the dysarthria was not totally attributable to cerebellar involvement 'some paralleled the components of spastic dysarthria'.

Assessment of dysarthria

The range, variability and degree of speech symptoms necessitate detailed and objective assessment in order to plan intervention and to monitor change. In some cases, clear description of the dysarthria can be of assistance in the medical diagnosis. There are several assessments of dysarthria available, including the methods described by Darley, Aronson and Brown (1975) and Enderby (1983). The latter comprises 11 sections, eight of which contain subtests administered by giving the patient a definitive task. The patient's response for each subtest is rated by the therapist on a 9-point rating scale which can be charted on a bargraph (see Figure 6.1). The sections include consideration of respiration, lips, jaw, palate, laryngeal, tongue, intelligibility, speaking rate, sensation and associated factors (e.g. posture, language).

The remissions and exacerbations of the disorder may well lead to variable performance, and certainly some patients may become almost anarthric and then recover the power of speech as their condition improves. Dysarthria may also vary as the result of fatigue. Lethargy and tiredness is experienced by many persons with MS even when they are only mildly affected and can result in reduced respiratory support, vocal amplitude and articulatory accuracy.

Patients may complain of these speech symptoms but may not demonstrate them at the time of being seen by the therapist. It can be helpful to ask the patient to make recordings of himself at intervals throughout the day if this is of concern.

Assessment of the dysarthria can be extended to include peak flow recordings, to assess respiratory support; nasalanemometry, to assess nasal emission; and electro-laryngography, to assess vocal cord performance. Furthermore, determination of environmental barriers that may interfere with communication should be part of all dysarthria evaluation and treatment: for example, to establish whether the patient is having trouble in certain situations such as meetings, telephone calls or noisy rooms.

Dysarthria therapy

It is unlikely that a patient with dysarthria associated with MS will return to being a normal speaker unless the dysarthric symptoms are temporary and associated with a lesion which recovers in remission. Most dysarthric speakers with this condition will slowly or intermittently deteriorate, the speed and extent of the deterioration relating to that of the disease itself. However, speech therapy has an active role to play and this role extends beyond the laudable palliative aspects of support and hope.

The main aim of speech therapy is to improve communication. This may lead to a primary emphasis on maximizing intelligibility or, if that

Figure 6.1 Frenchay Dysarthria Assessment. A completed example. Reproduced with permission from N.F.E.R. and Little Brown and Company.

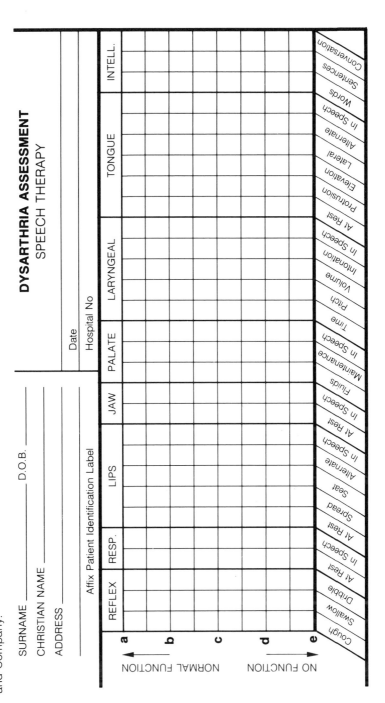

is already acceptable, then efforts at improving the quality and naturalness of communication may be appropriate.

The specific nature and type of treatment approaches available have increased in the last decade and this chapter cannot do full justice to them all. Therefore, treatment approaches for the most common of the speech symptoms will be described.

RESPIRATION/PHONATION

Poor respiratory support can lead to weak vocal quality, difficult speech and poor intonation and phrasing; after all, the respiratory system is the source of aerodynamic energy for speech. To a certain extent, respiration also has an effect on articulation; for example, sufficient air must be stopped and released for plosives (p,b,t,d) and sufficient air must be available to produce the friction in fricatives (f,v,sh).

It is not unusual to find that patients with MS have a weak trunk and poor posture and this can impede diaphragmatic excursion, thus adjusting posture is a prerequisite.

Diaphragmatic breathing exercises should use oral inhalation, emphasize controlled inspiration; the ability to hold the intake and slow expiration (or intermittent expiration) can be useful. The patient should, in this exercise as in others, be given clear guidance and objective goals so that he is encouraged to extend his ability. Introducing phonation with breathing can be used to extend control of expiration (say AH for as long as you can) or the power of expiration (say AH loudly then softly on the same breath). These exercises should lead to work on breath control for phrasing and contrastive stress. If the patient has limited respiratory reserve, improvements can be made by encouraging more frequent inhalations at appropriate times in the message. The patient should 'top up' his respiratory reserve rather than expending it all and then refilling.

Therapy for laryngeal function will differ according to whether the vocal quality suggests UMN, LMN or an ataxic disorder. Lesions of the vagus nerve can lead to a breathy vocal quality, hoarseness, a weak cough, low volume and low pitch. A 'spastic' voice tends to have a harsh, strangled quality with low pitch and volume. The phonation of patients with ataxia is often normal on prolonged vowel sound; however, in speech the voice may be overloud, have some vocal tremor and show inappropriate stress patterns. Laryngeal function is rarely treated in isolation and is usually treated with other speech aspects, particularly respiration. A patient with mild LMN involvement may well benefit from progressive exercises staged to extend the control and approximation of the vocal cords. Some of these exercises require vigour, energy and commitment; thus a frail patient may benefit more from being encouraged to use methods of speech conservation where over-articulation, pausing and phrasing can lead to more efficient use of the laryngeal function. The use of speech amplifiers may well be appropriate to ensure that communication is maintained and not avoided by the patient because of the effort involved.

The harsh quality associated with UMN phonation may be reduced by encouraging easy onset to voicing, and promoting generalized and specific relaxation techniques to reduce tone. A review of techniques to reduce hyperadduction and to increase airflow through the glottis is given by Prator and Swift (1984).

Appropriate laryngeal timing and modulation exercises may help the patient with an ataxic vocal quality. These exercises involve prompt initiation of phonation at the beginning of the exhalation phase of respiration (Yorkston, Beukelman and Bell, 1987; p.265) as this can reduce air wastage and fatigue during speech; and improvement of voice distinction between voiced and voiceless sounds, which is essential for intelligibility and improving the naturalness of speech. These tasks require a great deal of practice as they demand such accuracy of timing.

Usually, treatment of velopharyngeal dysfunction is only pursued directly if the nasal emission or hypernasality is out of line with other dysarthric components. This traditional hierarchy of treatment has been contested (Hardy, 1983; p.88; Netsell and Daniel, 1979) as there is the suggestion that efforts to improve other aspects of speech performance may not be effective if velopharyngeal function is not properly managed. For example, respiratory function and phonation are often compromised with dysarthria, and when this occurs along with poor velopharyngeal closure, then nasal escape will leave little intraoral pressure. Behavioural, prosthetic and surgical approaches have been advocated for the management of this deficiency (Yorkston, Beukelman and Bell, 1987). The former approach is more appropriate for patients with some residual function or where there is a likelihood of neurological improvement. The use of palatal lifts would be considered in the event that function is severely impaired and appears static. These appliances are usually made from acrylic and can either be attached to a denture as an extension or attached to a dental retainer. The lift is designed to elevate the soft palate so that it is kept in closer proximity to the nasopharyngeal wall (Enderby, Hathorn and Servant, 1984). This reduces the space to be closed when eating or producing oral sounds and has the added benefit of removing a sagging soft palate from the oral airway. Contraindications to a palatal lift include severe general dysarthria, poor cooperation and patients who are edentulous and have not tolerated a denture. Although palatal lifts can be used with dysarthria of different aetiologies, we have had striking success with some individuals with MS and would refute the suggestion that they are not suitable for those with degenerative disorders.

Respiration, phonation and velopharyngeal function are usually addressed prior to work on oral articulation being undertaken. The latter may be approached directly with strengthening and accuracy exercises, using biofeedback training with the aim of restoring techniques which camouflage the deficit to a greater or lesser extent.

Nearly all patients with dysarthria for whatever reason will be able to improve their articulation by becoming more focused, more deliberate and more realistic in their efforts. This requires the patient to monitor himself carefully and use techniques such as breaking words into syllables and adjusting movements to produce sounds in alternative ways. This, of course, takes insight and effort and patients may become fatigued and discouraged unless improvement is evident. It can be helpful to use charting techniques such as the one suggested by La Pointe (1979). This approach allows one to note change in any exercise defined precisely by the therapist. The amount of change expected would allow the therapist to adjust the exercises accordingly. Then, if little change is expected, easier tasks with lower goals would be appropriate.

Intelligibility drills involve the patient in attempting to articulate words which are similar except for a single phoneme. These can be useful as the patient's aim is to signal differences between the words to the listener and there is no prescribed way of achieving this. This allows the patient to adapt and adopt techniques of which he is capable with his residual function. The patient should be encouraged to educate his listeners to help with effective communication by listening carefully, improving eye contact, being close to the speaker, repeating and rephrasing, and the elimination of background noise.

When working with dysarthric speakers, especially those with MS, the therapist must be realistic; therefore, one of the strategies employed is that of identifying and repairing a breakdown in communication. The patient should be encouraged to realize when he has not made himself understood and should eventually know how to remedy the situation. This may lead the patient to know how to repeat himself in a way that is altered sufficiently to increase the likelihood of being comprehended, e.g. simplifying the sentence structure, choosing easier words, augmenting the communication with facial or hand gestures. In some cases, repairing communication may lead to the use of an alphabet board or other communication aid in order to facilitate and contain the interaction and these should be seen as appropriate augmentation of communication rather than 'failed oral speech'.

For patients who have occasional speaking difficulties, some general principles can be suggested. These include the importance of correct posture, encouraging relaxation, speaking slowly and with deliberate pauses, conserving energy by saying the most important points first when energy is greatest, speaking quietly and avoiding competing with background noise, and concentrating on articulation at certain times of the day.

DYSPHASIA

Dysphasia (both receptive and expressive) has been reported as being associated with exacerbations of MS. These patients may have severe word-finding problems, perseveration and use paraphasias and neologisms. The incidence of dysphasia with MS does not appear to have been studied and it is possible that more patients have high level dysphasic problems than have been recognized. It would seem appropriate that any patient with communication difficulty is screened to assess whether there is a concomitant language disorder even if this is not immediately apparent. Mild or moderate language disorders can lead to a patient misunderstanding more complex instructions, quick changes of subject, or nuances of meaning. Additionally, the patient may choose more simple sentence structures, tend to be repetitive, forget names and appear less willing to converse. One can imagine that these behaviours can be misinterpreted as the patient suffering generalized cognitive problems, personality changes or depression. Identification of the presence, type and degree of dysphasia will assist in more appropriate management which can only begin with a clear explanation of what a language disorder is to both the patient and the relatives.

In some cases, specific remediation to promote the use of residual language and to teach self-eliciting techniques can be useful. The value of applying speech therapy techniques used with stroke dysphasic patients to MS has not been fully explored.

However, with the patients who apparently suffer with this disorder where the lesion appears static or in remission, then one would speculate that specific speech therapy may be appropriate. Certainly, this distressing and perplexing symptom should be acknowledged and not confused with cognitive deficits by the patient, staff and relatives.

IMPAIRED COGNITION

Patients with relapsing or remitting MS were not found to be different from controls on measures of a broad range of cognitive and sensori-motor abilities, but 75% of chronic/progressive patients had cognitive deficits (Nelson *et al.,* 1982). Full psychometric assessment may be required and the results should be shared with the interdisciplinary team and family so that expectations are uniform and realistic. Patients with mild problems may benefit from being taught rehearsal strategies, how to use visual and auditory imagery or word association, encouraged to make lists, preplan, and should be allowed plenty of time even for simple tasks. This is dealt with in more detail elsewhere in the book.

MUTISM

A few patients have demonstrated periods of mutism. In my experience, these periods have been temporary. It has been difficult to establish whether these periods of complete inability and apparent unwillingness to communicate in any way are related to a specific lesion (for example, in the frontal lobe) or due to a psychiatric or psychological condition. One patient, having recovered from a period of mutism, reported feelings and experiences which I felt were similar to an extreme apraxia affecting more than the oro-motor system.

DEAFNESS

Decreased hearing associated with MS has been mentioned in several studies. Merritt's (1979; p.782) review suggests a frequency of 6%. However, this is likely to include many with a coincidental hearing problem. Quire, Regan and Murray (1984) suggest that a specific hearing problem can be detected in some MS patients and this particular problem was not related to a peripheral origin. They report that some patients are specifically 'deaf' to changes in 'tone pitch' even when auditory sensitivity is not impaired. Frequency shift deafness can be understood in terms of the concept that the auditory pathway contains separate neural mechanisms sensitive to changes in the intensity and pitch of a tone. It has been suggested that patients with degraded ability to hear changes in tone pitch might, as a result, have abnormal speech comprehension problems, although they may have a normal audiogram.

LOSS OF EMOTIONAL CONTROL

Patients with MS may experience loss of control of the expression of emotions. Pseudobulbar laughing and crying may be associated with spastic bulbar dysfunction and dysarthria and is thought to be a product of muscular spasm or increased tone rather than a change in actual mood. However, if a patient is unable to inhibit an inappropriate emotional response, such as false laughter or crying, this may lead to anger or frustration leading to real tears. Pseudobulbar laughing must not be confused with euphoria; the latter involves actual mood changes or swings which can result from certain organic lesions leading the patient to be euphoric or labile. These responses can be exasperating and perplexing to patients and relatives and, whilst no specific treatment seems particularly efficacious, it is important to explain the nature of the dysfunction so at least it is recognized. Frequently, the approach is to play down the emotional expression when it occurs and use a distractor to give the patient time to recover.

DEPRESSION

The emotional impact of MS on patients can be devastating, leading to an understandable state of depression. This may be a reaction to loss of function and uncertainty of the future and can lead to lethargy, sluggishness and social withdrawal. A patient may function at a level lower than that of which he is capable, find difficulty in being motivated and learning or retaining information. Depression can be mistaken as fatigue or cognitive deficits and can make any communication disorder worse as the patient may well become less willing to interact both verbally and non-verbally. Suicidal tendencies are frequently present (Langworthy, 1948; Surridge, 1969; Weinstein, 1970; Schwartz and Perron, 1972) as life can be perceived as having no hope. If a patient is this depressed, efforts at rehabilitation can be futile until the mood is improved and, whilst antidepressants and tranquilizers may have a role, support and counselling by an appropriate professional may assist with the patient coming to terms with his problems and resolving some anxieties.

DYSPHAGIA

There are many reasons why a patient may complain of problems with eating and drinking. Obviously, the management of a dysphagic difficulty relating to a weak tongue and resulting in poor control of the bolus is different from that of dysphagia caused by a sluggish swallow reflex. It is therefore essential to establish the nature of the dysphagia and its underlying cause before attempting to intervene. Detailed history taking, observation and specific dysphagia assessment are needed with any patient complaining of dysphagia. Videofluoroscopy can be useful in some instances. Varying degrees of swallowing difficulty may occur in patients with MS. Again, remissions and exacerbation of dysphagic symptoms are common but longstanding severe swallowing problems are usually only found in the chronically disabled patient. The underlying neurological lesion may affect one or multiple cranial nerves, the upper motor neurones and/or the cortex and cerebellum. In a study of 75 MS patients, a reduction in pharyngeal peristalsis and delayed swallow reflex were the most common dysphagic problems (Logemann, 1983).

Oral phase disorders

If the hypoglossal nerve (X) is affected, the patient's lingual control of bolus manipulation will be affected. Facial nerve (VII) involvement will result in poor lip seal and lead to drooling and may affect the sense of taste.

The trigeminal nerve (V) is responsible for motor innervation of the masseter and deficits can lead to a weak chew. Oral phase difficulties can be assisted by changing the consistency of the diet, altering posture and teaching the patient a routine for swallowing to make it more purposeful.

82

Pharyngeal phase

The swallow reflex and pharyngeal peristalsis may be reduced if the tenth cranial nerve is affected, rendering swallowing slow and difficult. Involvement of the vagus will lead to poor laryngeal function and airway protection will be reduced. There will be a weak, ineffective cough which can result in aspiration. Logemann (1983) has described techniques which may assist, including thermal stimulation of the fauces. The summary in this chapter gives only a brief explanation of possible dysphagic disorders and readers are recommended to turn to Groher (1984) for more detail.

Dysphagia management

'Treatment of dysphagia in MS focuses on the patient's environment, body position, style of eating and types of food eaten' (Ruttenberg, 1985). First of all it is important for the patient and his carer to appreciate the nature of the problem. Reducing anxiety can lessen the problem as the patient will be more relaxed, giving improved muscle control and assisting him/her to compensate. Verbal cues and 'thinking about swallowing' can facilitate cortical control. Patients should be encouraged to take their time and distractions should be reduced.

If the patient becomes fatigued with the effort of eating, it is advisable to have small frequent meals with an easy texture. The use of food supplements and advice from the dietitian should be considered before the patient becomes debilitated, as general weakness from under-eating can lead to a vicious circle in the condition. As aspiration is more likely when the patient is tired, it may be necessary to feed the patient if this reduces the effort and allows oral feeding to be continued.

The patient's posture is crucial and mild dysphagic problems can be eliminated with simple alterations. The back should be straight and head slightly flexed, which will allow the bolus to enter the pharynx more easily whilst the back of the tongue is assisting the protection of the airway.

If the patient is choking regularly the carers should be taught the appropriate methods of managing choking, and a sucker should be provided.

Some MS patients will have intermittent dysphagic episodes related to exacerbations of the condition. It may be necessary to feed via a nasogastric tube to prevent further decline until the general condition improves. We have had experience of a few patients requiring intermittent tube feeding to help regain weight and stamina, which improves the general medical condition, which in turn improves the dysphagia.

Alternative methods of feeding should be considered if feeding becomes so laborious that it is no longer practicable, aspiration pneumonia becomes a repetitive event, the patient loses weight severely and continually, or in the event of severe dehydration.

Nasogastric feeding, using a small-bore tube which does not require frequent changing, may relieve both the patient and relatives, although reluctance is not unusual. Occasionally, surgical placement of a feeding tube may be warranted, the most common procedure being oesophagostomy, gastrostomy and jejunostomy.

DEHYDRATION

MS patients are at particular risk of becoming dehydrated which can lead to medical and cognitive problems, along with the danger of kindling a relapse. Frequently, drinking is more difficult than eating solids. This can be because it is easier to spill with an ataxic tremor. Drinks dribble from the mouth more readily and tend to escape into the airway more easily leading to choking. Furthermore, bladder problems or difficulty in getting to the toilet may lead to the patient purposefully deciding to reduce liquid intake. Particular notice and encouragement should be given to hydration.

ANOREXIA

Some patients may have perceptions and behaviours similar to anorexia. They may consciously or sub-consciously reduce food intake; this may be a stress reaction, or related to concerns that their weight might be a burden on carers, or it may be an effort to remain childlike. The problems may mimic dysphagia or compound dysphagia and the therapist should be alert to these possibilities.

COMMUNICATION AIDS

The numbers of patients with MS who would benefit from a communication aid, either permanently or occasionally, is hard to
establish. The numbers appear small but it is likely that some
patients who would be helped in this may not have been referred for
such an assessment. This may be because of the low expectations
reached when the disorder is chronic and progressive. Additionally,
the medical practitioner may not have considered communication as
possible or necessary as the problem is insidious in nature.

There are a great variety of communication aids, which range
from simple alphabet charts and word boards to sophisticated
appliances with microprocessors and digitized speech. No one aid
can be viewed as best. Each person's needs and abilities along with
environmental constraints have to be assessed and only then will it
become evident whether a certain approach would be appropriate.
There are a number of Communication Aid Centres throughout the
United Kingdom. The staff will not only arrange for assessment and
assist with acquiring the chosen equipment, but will frequently
modify any switches and teach the user the strategies to use for
effective communication with an aid.

Some persons with MS will require an aid to augment speech,
others will require an aid to replace speech. The former may require
an amplifier or an aid to use when they are fatigued, whilst the latter
may depend on a system as their only method of communication. It
is often useful to introduce a communication system to the patient
when it is only needed as a back-up, e.g. if the patient's speech is
difficult to understand in a noisy environment. The aid can then be
introduced to help in a specific situation and if found to be beneficial
the patient will turn to it naturally as, or if, speech deteriorates
further.

The most common causes of communication aids being under-used
are related to inappropriate equipment being provided following
inadequate assessment, or if the patient and carer are not given sufficient training and practice in its use. The patient with a communication system should be reviewed regularly so that changes in needs
and status are responded to (Enderby, 1987).

The communication impairments of persons with MS should be
viewed as a challenge to the speech therapist. Appropriate assessment
and clear detection of the underlying pathology is certainly more
complex in this disorder than in many others. Transient and changing
symptomology, cognitive, sensory motoric and psychological

impairments, demand skills and persistence if the therapist is to play a full part in assisting the patient in understanding and tackling this disease.

REFERENCES

Beukelman, D.R., Kraft, G. and Freal, J. (1985) Expressive communication disorders in persons with multiple sclerosis: A survey. *Archives of Physical Medicine and Rehabilitation,* **66**, 675-7.

Charcot, J. (1877) *Lecture on Diseases of the Nervous System.* New Sydenham Society, London.

Darley, F.L., Aronson, A.E. and Brown, J.R. (1969) Differential diagnostic patterns of dysarthria. *Journal of Speech and Hearing Research,* **12**, 246-69.

Darley, F.L., Aronson, A.E. and Brown, J.R. (1975) *Motor Speech Disorders.* W.B. Saunders, Philadelphia.

Darley, F.L., Brown, J.R. and Goldstein, N.P. (1972) Dysarthria in multiple sclerosis. *Journal of Speech and Hearing Research,* **15**, 229-45.

Enderby, P.M. (1983) *Frenchay Dysarthria Assessment.* College-Hill Press, San Diego.

Enderby, P., Hathorn, I. and Servant, S. (1984) The use of intra-oral appliances in the management of acquired velopharyngeal disorders. *British Dental Journal,* Sept., 157-60.

Enderby, P. (1987) *Assistive Communication Aids for the Speech Impaired.* Churchill Livingstone, Edinburgh.

Groher, M.E. (1984) *Dysphagia. Diagnosis and Management.* Butterworths, Boston.

Hardy, J. (1983) *Cerebral Palsy.* Prentice Hall, Englewood Cliffs N.J., p.88.

Ivers, R. and Goldstein, N. (1963) Multiple sclerosis: A current appraisal of symptoms and signs. *Proceedings of the Staff of Meetings of the Mayo Clinic,* **38**, 457-66.

Kurtzke, J.F. (1983) Epidemiology of multiple sclerosis, in J.F. Hallpike, C.W.M. Adams and W.W. Tourtellotte (eds) Multiple Sclerosis, pathology, diagnosis and management. Chapman and Hall, London, ch.3, pp. 47-95.

Langworthy, O. (1948) Relation of personality problems to onset and progress of multiple sclerosis. *Archives Neurology and Psychiatry,* **59**, 13.

La Pointe, L.L. (1979) *Base 10 Response Form.* C.C. Publications Ltd., Oregon.

Logemann, J. (1983) *Evaluation and Treatment of Swallowing Disorders.* College-Hill Press, Boston.

Merritt, H.H. (1979) *A Text Book of Neurology.* Lea and Febiger.

Nelson, L.M., Thompson, D.S. and Heaton, R.H. (1982) Cognitive deficits in multiple sclerosis. *Society for Neurosciences Abstracts,* **8** (2), 629.

Netsell, R. and Daniel, B. (1979) Dysarthria in adults: Physiologic approach to rehabilitation. *Archives of Physical Medicine and Rehabilitation,* **60**, 502-8.

Prator, R.J. and Swift, R.W. (1984) *Manual of Voice Therapy*. Little, Brown and Co., Boston.

Quire, D.B., Regan, D. and Murray, T.J. (1984) Degraded discrimination between speech-like sounds by patients with multiple sclerosis and Freidrichs ataxia. *Brain*, **107**, 113–22.

Ruttenberg, N. (1985) Assessment and treatment of speech and swallowing problems in patients with multiple sclerosis, in *Interdisciplinary Rehabilitation of Multiple Sclerosis and Neuromuscular Disorders* (eds F, Maloney, J. Burk and S. Ringel). J.B. Lippincott Co., Philadelphia.

Schwartz, M.L. and Perron, M. (1972) Suicide and fatal accidents in multiple sclerosis. *Omega*, **3**, 291–3.

Surridge, D. (1969) An investigation into some aspects of multiple sclerosis. *British Journal of Psychiatry*, **115**, 749–64.

Weinstein, E.A. (1970) Behavioural aspects of multiple sclerosis. *Modern Treatment*, **7**, 961–8.

Yorkston, K.M., Beukelman, D.R. and Bell, K.R. (1987) *Clinical Management of Dysarthric Speakers*. Taylor and Francis, London.

7

Counselling

Julia Segal

Multiple sclerosis (MS) affects people emotionally as well as physically. Existing difficulties with relationships, social functioning and thinking or feeling may be exacerbated by the MS. Even before MS causes practical problems it can cause enormous emotional turmoil. Segal (1986) and Robinson (1988) have described some of these reactions. As Grant *et al.* have shown (1989), many people diagnosed with MS have suffered severe disturbances in their lives in the months previous to onset of symptoms. How people react to these difficulties can be of vital importance for their whole lives.

Even where the MS itself gets worse, emotionally people can get better, particularly with counselling. This can off-set the gloom and hopelessness of the medical picture. Counsellors can help people find their own ways to change many aspects of their lives, with consequent improvements in their thoughts, feelings and social relationships.

In Britain, unlike the United States, counselling has not in the past been offered as a matter of course to people with MS or any other life-threatening disease. The general practitioner has been seen as the main source of advice on how to cope, with back-up provided by nurses and social workers. Approaches to counsellors tend to be made in a context which implies some kind of 'failure to cope'. This situation may change in the future. One recommendation is that a consultation with a counsellor should be automatic for anyone with MS or who lives with someone who has it.

WHY OFFER COUNSELLING?

Counselling offers people an opportunity to reflect upon and think about their lives. A good counsellor helps people to look at the changes the MS has brought into their lives and to grieve for their losses. MS brings many losses of subtle kinds, such as loss of hopes or expectations, as well as the more obvious ones (Burnfield, 1985).

'I've never been able to bear the idea of being dependent on other people.'
'My husband is no longer the supportive, responsible partner I married.'
'I know I'm going to die soon, so what is the point of doing anything?'

With help people come to distinguish what they have actually lost from what they are afraid they have lost or do not have to lose.

'I've lost everything . . . well, no, of course my wife won't leave me . . . no, I haven't actually lost my job, they are keeping me on though I don't really do much . . . yes, the children seem OK . . . I get bad-tempered with them when I can't do something . . .'

For the man who said this there were very real losses which needed to be acknowledged, including a loss of self-respect. These were different from the losses he thought he had to bear.

In the counselling room people have the opportunity to examine thoughts and feelings which they would not dare have outside. Secret, often terrifying ideas can be explored and when they are shared with the counsellor they may be changed. Often they turn out to be unrealistic. For example:

'If I allow myself to have negative thoughts my MS will get worse.'
'I am going to die in a couple of years and I shall never see my children grow up.'

In both these cases, once examined these ideas appeared quite unrealistic to the people concerned.

Professional counsellors are in a different position from people offering a more informal 'listening ear'. Some of the anxieties involved can only be shared with someone who is not in a position to act upon them or carelessly pass them on to anyone else. For example:

'I sometimes hate him so much I don't care what happens to him: I just want to walk out and never come back.'
'I sometimes hit my children really hard . . . My father used to beat me . . . I'm afraid of what I'll do to them . . .'

ANXIETIES RAISED BY MS

MS seems to raise anxieties which already existed for the people concerned. People often read into it their worst fears. This means that everyone reacts differently; what is important for one person with MS is not so important for another. Counsellors are generally skilled in discovering what MS means to the individual and family, rather than in predicting what will concern them. This is important, particularly where the experience of being diagnosed MS has included a helplessness and powerlessness, and a sense that nobody is really interested.

IS IT ALL IN THE MIND?

Where the diagnosis has been questionable for a long time, people may have wondered 'how much is it in the mind?' (Robinson, 1988; p.31). For those with a fear or experience of mental illness this can be very disturbing, while for others it seems of little consequence. Part of the issue here is whether the MS can be cured by 'mind over matter' (Robinson, 1988; pp. 98–9). If it is misdiagnosed hysteria, there is hope in that psychotherapy or time might cure it. On the other hand, some people are more afraid of being mad than of being physically ill. The difficulty for anyone, be they patient, doctor or relative, is differentiating between MS, conversion hysteria or 'laziness'. The relevant issue is what the person and their family believe because what doctors and other professionals say is often selectively perceived to fit in with these beliefs.

WHAT CAUSED THE MS?

Many people are anxious about what they or someone else did to cause the MS (Helman, 1984; p.75). They often have quite unreasonable 'explanations' which need to be examined. For example:

'They don't know do they . . . I think she has it because I had a virus when I was six months pregnant with her . . .'
'I feel I brought it on myself; I was actually relieved to be ill, and not to have to worry about work any more; I feel I must have somehow caused it in order to get out of the situation I was in.'

Often people watch themselves carefully to discover what effect their behaviour has on the MS. A professional may have a useful role helping to distinguish between behaviour which might make the MS worse and behaviour which is unlikely to.

OLD SYMPTOMS SHOWING UP VERSUS THE MS GETTING WORSE

People may need to be told the difference between symptoms showing up and the MS getting worse. Old symptoms often recur after exercise, or when the person is hot or tired or emotional (Hewer, 1980). This is not the same as new symptoms developing. Where people are trying to forget the MS, recurrence of old symptoms reminds them it has not gone away. Their emotional state at this point then depends on their automatic, unthinking fears and anxieties connected with the MS. If these have been thought about and made bearable, recurrent symptoms may be more easily tolerated from an emotional point of view. Where the fears are still in a primitive, unthought-out state, there may be emotional reactions which reflect panic about what will happen if the MS does not go away. There may be outbursts which appear quite out of proportion to the apparent situation, or the person may withdraw, or become suddenly anxious about something apparently quite unconnected.

FEAR OF MAKING THE MS WORSE

Family dynamics can be affected by fear of making the MS worse. Family life can be made intolerable if people are scared of being upset or of upsetting the person with MS in case it gets worse. This is an important point where children are concerned. They frequently seem to feel that their behaviour or thoughts can make their parent's MS better or worse. The level of anxiety and consequent difficulty this creates in families cannot be overestimated.

SEX

Man with MS: 'Sex is no problem: I gave it up; it made me worse.'
Counsellor: 'What does your wife think of that?'
Man: 'I don't know, I haven't asked her.'

91

Sexual relationships can be affected by MS in many ways. Full or partial loss of erection may be an early symptom, and when it is not recognized as part of MS, sexual relationships may be threatened. Both men and women can be affected by loss of sensation as well as by worries, resentments and anxieties connected with MS. There can also be loss of drive and enthusiasm which may have both emotional and physical origins.

Relationships may also be affected by practical issues such as incontinence or severe spasms, both of which sometimes lead couples to sleep apart for the first time. This in turn can reduce the amount of non-sexual physical contact and closeness. Previous difficulties and anxieties around sex may be exacerbated and specialist sexual or marital counselling may be helpful.

Relationship difficulties cause many couples to seek to discover what is due to the MS and what to their personalities, in order to know whether to make allowances or not. It is difficult, if not impossible, in most cases to do this with any degree of certainty. The question of making allowances is in itself something which may be usefully discussed. The rights and duties of couples towards each other have to be modified by illness, but a chronic illness is very different from a short-term one and the 'normal' allowances made for ill people may not be appropriate, therefore what should and should not be tolerated may have to be negotiated.

LOSS OF ROLE

Family life may also be seriously affected if the parent with MS abdicates responsibility for parenting. Both men and women sometimes seem to put all their energy into maintaining their job to the extent of neglecting their roles as partner and parent. When MS is added to this situation real problems may be caused for all the family. Sometimes attempts to protect a parent with MS from stress can remove them from family decision making and support-giving. Children and spouses may hesitate to show their distress at this for fear of making things worse; this can mean that changes which could be made are not considered.

An 11-year-old girl – with no obvious problems – did not tell her mother about falling out with her best friend at school because 'granny said I wasn't to upset her'. She told the counsellor her grandmother and her father had both told her that the mother's MS would get worse if she upset her. This was particularly sad for the family because her mother was unable to do much for her daughter physically, but she was a good listener and the role of 'supportive mum' was one she could have fulfilled better than most.

UNCERTAINTY

MS leaves people with many questions and doubts (Wright, 1983; p.109; Robinson, 1988; pp. 36–40). How long will it remain the way it is now? How bad will it get? How soon before another attack, and will it be like the last one? When and how will I die? What caused it? What am I doing now that will make it worse – can I do anything to improve my chances? Am I trying as hard as I can? Should I be trying harder or should I be allowing myself to rest? Should I 'accept' or 'fight' the MS?

Uncertainty seems to be very hard to bear. One temptation is to ignore all these questions and some people keep themselves busy in order not to think about them. Sometimes this is because they are sure they know the answers.

One woman's insistence that 'I don't think about it . . .' was covering a conviction that 'it' was 'the end', which meant a horrible, lonely death in a crowded ward. She had kept this idea quite separate from an equally strong conviction that her boyfriend would be with her to the end. Encouragement to think about it with the counsellor enabled this woman to put the two ideas together, with other information she already possessed, in a way which left her far less frightened.

It can be useful to help people to hold onto the fact that these questions are unanswerable, and that the various possibilities, their consequences and the anxieties about them, can be discussed. Many of these questions may be stated as 'either/or' when in fact it may be more appropriate to consider them as 'both/and'. This is not easy and requires that the counsellor can face very distressing thoughts.

A woman was very angry that her husband who had MS forgot to ask how she had got on at a hospital appointment. With the counsellor the couple looked at the possibility that his memory had been affected by the MS. They found this very painful indeed and it was an idea that they had resisted for a long time. Together they also looked at the possibility that the husband had forgotten for other reasons to do with the relationship. The wife felt that 'really' he wanted all the attention himself and was jealous of her being ill too. The counsellor added other possibilities: perhaps he wanted her to feel nobody was interested in her, as he felt no-one was really interested in him; but perhaps too he was afraid it was his fault she was in pain, and wanted to blot out all thoughts of it. These were all feelings the wife shared with her husband. She was jealous of the attention he received from his mother when she had none, and she felt the MS was her fault and that no-one was interested in her. Becoming aware of the extent to which they shared the difficult feelings seemed to enable them to live together less acrimoniously.

CONTROL

One reason why uncertainty is so unbearable is because it seems to take away a sense of being in control of one's life. Looking at this can uncover illusions (Segal, 1987).

For one young woman, being in control meant to her keeping the respect of her father, and also keeping her husband, because she felt she had made him love her. Throwing doubt on the power she had exerted over him enabled her to question her need to be in control so much.

INDEPENDENCE

A related issue is that of independence. People often say they fear the loss of their independence (Cunningham, 1977; pp. 59–63; Wright, 1983). What they mean by this is different for each individual, and exploring it in counselling can change their view. It is often used as a blanket term, when it can be usefully broken down.

Sue: 'I'd hate the wheelchair; I think it's the loss of independence . . .'
Counsellor: 'In what way do you mean?'
Sue: 'Well, . . . not being able to get out.'

Further exploration revealed that Sue had recently succeeded in getting out of a disastrous marriage and for her 'independence' meant escape from an intolerable relationship. Clarifying this enabled her to think afresh about what the wheelchair would or would not prevent.

The idea of 'independence' sometimes seems to be developed as an ideal in childhood as a reaction to the idea of being dependent upon unreliable or uncontrollable adults. Fears of losing independence may be related then to fears of being faced with feeling again like a miserable, dependent child whose needs are not being met. Pretending to be an adult may at the time have seemed the only way to survive and in adulthood the ability to ask for help may never have been developed. MS may force the issue with a threat of considerable emotional pain and very conflicting feelings (Robinson, 1988; p.68).

Real experiences of being dependent upon unsatisfactory nurses or doctors can also contribute to fears of being dependent. For example:

'I was in hospital . . . I wanted a bedpan and the nurses kept saying "hold on a minute . . ." I couldn't, but they didn't seem to realize; this one nurse, she really shouted at me, "couldn't you have waited just a minute?" . . .'

Many professionals also idealize 'independence' and fail to recognize that emotional dependence is a necessary part of any love relationship. Failure to acknowledge the value of adult forms of interdependence can make living with MS harder (Segal, 1987).

FEELING BAD

Without quite realizing it, people often seem to confuse being bad physically with being a bad person. There can be some reality in this, since illness generally makes people self-centred, often bad-tempered, and difficult to live with. The guilt of behaving in unacceptable ways adds to the difficulty of the MS. The fear that such 'badness' is somehow contagious may give rise to the belief that the only solution is to separate the person with MS from other family members by isolating them, or by somebody leaving home. Anxieties about being worthy of being loved are also part of this and can adversely affect all the family.

ANGER

Many people, but not all, react with anger (Robinson, 1983). Those with MS can be angry with the MS, with their own bodies or with someone they blame for the situation.

'I get really angry with my legs when they won't work; I shout at them . . .'
'All I ask is that I should get back the use of my legs . . . I don't feel that is unreasonable.'

The young man saying this did not believe in God, but he did seem to feel that someone had power over his MS.

Not only family members but also professionals can get angry with the person who has MS, perhaps for having it, perhaps for the way they are reacting to it.

'I could put up with the MS but I can't stand his negative attitude.'

Often attempts to hide the anger cause trouble within families, where tensions build up to breaking point because nobody wants to confess to being angry.

GUILT

Guilt is closely connected with anger. People frequently feel guilty about being angry, just as they feel guilty about being ill. They may feel guilty about the way they are handling their MS, or guilty about the way they are causing difficulties for others because of the MS, or even guilty about their own supposed badness of their failure or their impotence. Relatives and professionals who do not have MS can feel guilty towards people who have it. An example is:

'When the sun is shining and I feel happy then I suddenly think, how can I be happy when my daughter has MS? I must be a terrible mother. I should be wishing I had it instead of her, but I don't.'

Where people feel too guilty, they may develop an appearance of not caring any more.

Relatives, particularly children, often feel guilty that they have failed to make the person they love better. They may feel, without realizing it, that if their love was stronger, the person with MS would get better. This can shake their belief in their own goodness, and for children is a serious attack on their self-perception.

Professionals may also feel guilty that their interventions have not helped, as well as angry that their treatment has be interrupted by the MS. For example, an experienced physiotherapist said:

'I felt really guilty when she had a relapse; I kept thinking – what did I do wrong? I knew it was nothing to do with what I did, but I still felt it. I got over it when she got better. Then I felt angry – why did she have a relapse? It's all her fault, she's ruined my treatment plan.'

VERBAL AND NON-VERBAL COMMUNICATION

Many people have difficulty putting their thoughts, needs, wishes and longings into words. 'Society' or close relatives may be attacked: 'if they really cared they would understand without being told'. Partners, children or professionals may struggle with increasing frustration to guess what is required, when the non-verbal messages are powerful but ambiguous. Counselling can sometimes assist in the development of more verbal communication. This makes life with MS easier, particularly if the assistance of other people is necessary at times.

INFORMAL COUNSELLING

Much of the informal advice given to people with MS seems to come from doctors. Some is seen by patients as very helpful. For example:

'I am afraid I only have two other patients with MS; we're going to have to find out about it together.'
'Come and talk to me again next week when you've had time to think about it.'

Other advice may be far from helpful:

'Perhaps you should think about getting sterilized.'

Some advice may be completely unrealistic:

'You should go away and not think about it, just carry on as normal.'
'Tell me what you want from me.'

Listening to people

Many professional health workers have an idea that listening to people is supposed to be helpful, without really believing that this can be so. They may feel they should somehow steer the conversation in positive directions, or that they should have something to offer. It is seldom fully recognized that paying attention, listening intelligently and having someone else acknowledge reality, both good and bad, is always in some way a relief. Sometimes where it is recognized, people become scared of the power this has to create a relationship where they may not want one. They may prefer to take an approach which keeps all negative thoughts and all real human contact at bay.

Should I listen?

Many professionals find themselves in a position where they feel someone with MS, or their partner or a member of the family needs someone to talk to. They have to decide if they are prepared to take the time to listen or not. Some feel they do not know enough to start, or are annoyed by the demands made on them. Some feel guilty about taking the time off their real job to listen when they feel they cannot really help, even though they are also aware that they cannot work with a patient who is too preoccupied with other troubles.

Choosing not to listen

Professionals may have neither the time, the training, the inclination nor the support necessary to listen to people with MS who may want to talk about harrowing experiences. Some decide not to make any space for allowing people to talk about themselves. Others simply prevent the person talking without having made a conscious decision to do so. Some try to find a compromise, whereby they listen briefly and then steer the conversation back. These kinds of issues can determine whether a patient is offered further appointments or not.

With any of these strategies, some professionals feel guilty about the times they refuse to listen, while others recognize their own limitations and the fact that they cannot help everyone.

Where there is a counsellor to whom the patient can be referred, the problem may be lessened. A counsellor can also sometimes help the professional with their own feelings about the patient concerned. When there has been a very demanding or disturbing interaction between patient and professional a counsellor's help may enable the professional to continue to offer a limited amount of sensitive listening.

Sometimes discussion with colleagues can help clarify the

professional's own realistic and unrealistic beliefs about their capacity.

Choosing to listen

Some professionals do allow people to talk about their feelings or experiences connected with the MS, or about their lives in general.

Here they have to make certain decisions, such as 'how far to get involved'; such decisions will be made in the light of experience. The attitude of colleagues will also be important. Many recognize that boundaries of some kind have to be held. It is where and how to draw these boundaries which is often difficult.

Disturbing nature of others' emotions

The impact of other people's emotions can be at times extremely disturbing. There seem to be some people who disturb everyone they meet. Others hit a particular raw nerve for one person, without affecting others in the same way.

Professional counsellors have to be in supervision with an experienced colleague, and such supervision helps to maintain the ability to listen without being traumatized by others' problems. Anyone indulging in informal counselling should be prepared to find a professional counsellor who is able to offer them assistance in this way, and thereby reduce the many risks involved.

Interference with the primary task

Sometimes listening to patients' problems prevents professional health workers from doing the job for which they are trained. If this is happening for much of the time, it may reflect or cause dissatisfaction with the work. If a counsellor or social worker is needed to enable the other professionals to do their jobs, it might be preferable to arrange for routine referral, rather than depriving patients of therapy by giving unskilled counselling instead.

Over a period of time the kind, listening nurse, dietitian or physiotherapist may become gradually more short-tempered and impatient with other peoples' troubles. Even one bad experience may leave the professional vowing never to listen to a patient again.

There are people who have a peculiar capacity to draw in anyone who offers a listening ear, and then systematically to set about destroying their self-confidence, belief in themselves and their ability to work. Becoming involved with this kind of person can permanently or temporarily destroy the professionals' willingness to offer an informal listening ear to anyone.

Defences evolved by professional counsellors against this kind of behaviour include the strict boundaries of time and place for the counselling session, and strict boundaries of role for the counsellor. It may or may not be possible to adapt these for use in more informal settings.

Cruelty

Cruel physical and verbal attacks are not uncommon in households where someone has a chronic illness and professionals are not immune to becoming cruel themselves. Nurses are particularly vulnerable, as their job allows them all kinds of covert means of hurting or humiliating patients. Where they find themselves, or colleagues, doing this, their own self-respect may be severely threatened and they may have great difficulty in confessing even to the impulse to hurt. Since they do not manage to share their guilt, they may never receive any help in understanding what went on and so preventing it happening again. It is becoming known, for example, that those who have been abused as children may put enormous pressure on others to repeat the abuse; the effect of this where it succeeds with a professional can be devastating (Sinason, 1988).

Home visiting

One of the issues which arises with counselling people with severe disabilities is the question of whether to attempt to offer counselling at home. This needs to be considered carefully. There are usually plenty of organizations, voluntary and statutory, which can provide transport for people with disabilities. Sometimes effort by the client to find transport can lead to an opening up of opportunities for social contact, for shopping trips, and a new involvement in the community. Clearly there are people who cannot be moved, and getting out is enormously difficult for some people, but the gains can be considerable.

One of the difficulties of being disabled is the way other people treat disabled people as pitiable and as 'different' from others in ways in which they are not necessarily any different at all. It is difficult for most people to make the effort to go for counselling or psychotherapy and excuses will be made to put it off, perhaps for many years. Counselling involves painful work by the counsellee, and one of the few ways in which the counsellor can be sure they have permission to say the unpalatable things they must say is that the person involved has decided to attend.

Much of the communication between counsellee and counsellor is non-verbal. The counsellor makes important 'statements' by being available at certain times in an entirely trustworthy fashion and the counsellee can leave, fail to turn up to a session or turn up late. There are non-verbal messages which can be conveyed, by failing to answer the door to a counsellor, or by ways of handling other visitors, but these may cause the counsellee far more difficulty than simply 'forgetting' to turn up for an appointment.

Against this, or course, is the fact that there are real transport problems for people with MS and it is part and parcel of the state of being dependent upon others that appointments may not be kept as they would be if the person were dependent only on their own mobility. As such, this is a topic which can be usefully discussed in counselling. Punctuality is just as much a legitimate topic within counselling people with MS as it is for anyone else, and discovering some of the difficulties in keeping appointments, or in persuading others to be punctual, can open up questions about the amount of control which the person with MS in fact has. Some turn out to have rather more than might be imagined, and the discussion may lead on to a new discovery of ways of making helpers more amenable. The central issue of control of others and the self comes alive within the counselling.

There are further problems involved when a counsellor visits a counsellee at home. The person is trapped in that what they have to say remains 'in the room' and cannot be 'left behind' if they so wish, when they leave. The counsellor and counsellee must be more careful about what is revealed, and the power of the work is reduced.

Both counsellee's and counsellor's minds and attention are also likely to be distracted in a house which is not set up for private counselling sessions. Listening for door-bells, children, spouses, or telephones may all reduce the attention of the counsellor for the person's conscious and unconscious communication which requires understanding. The counsellee, rather than the counsellor, must hold the responsibility for keeping other people out of the session, and this can cause distractions.

In these ways the person who is visited at home is deprived of the standard and quality of counselling offered to people who are not disabled or ill. There may be times when the decision is made to offer home counselling sessions, but the loss to the counsellee of the opportunity for 'normal' counselling may need to be discussed in the sessions.

CONCLUSION

This chapter has looked at some aspects of counselling people with MS in a formal or an informal setting. Relations between the person with MS and the professional who has to decide whether or not to listen have been discussed, as well as some of the issues which arise when people think about the effect of MS on their lives.

REFERENCES

Burnfield, A. (1985) *Multiple Sclerosis: A personal exploration.* Souvenir Press, London.

Cunningham, D.J. (1977) Stigma and social isolation: self-perceived problems of a group of multiple sclerosis sufferers. Report No.27. Health Services Research Unit, Centre for Research in the Social Services, University of Kent, Canterbury.

Grant, I., Brown, G.W., Harris, T. *et al.* (1989) Severely threatening events and marked life difficulties preceding onset or exacerbation of multiple sclerosis. *Journal of Neurology, Neurosurgery and Psychiatry,* **52**, 8–13.

Helman, C. (1984) *Culture, Health and Illness.* Wright, Bristol.

Hewer, R.L. (1980) Multiple sclerosis management and rehabilitation. *International Rehabilitation Medicine,* **2**, 116–25.

Robinson, I. (1983) Discovering the diagnosis of MS. General Report No.3, Brunel-ARMS Research Unit, Dept. Human Sciences, Brunel, University of W. London.

Robinson, I. (1988) *Multiple Sclerosis.* Routledge, London.

Segal, J.C. (1986) *Emotional Reactions to MS.* ARMS publication.

Segal, J.C. (1987) Independence and Control: Issues in the counselling of people with MS. *Counselling,* No.62, 10–17.

Sinason, V. (1988) Smiling, swallowing, sickening and stupefying: the effect of sexual abuse on the child. *Psychoanalytic Psychotherapy,* **3**(2), 97–111.

Wright, B.A. (1983) *Physical Disability: A psychosocial approach* (2nd edn). Harper and Row, New York.

8

Nutrition

Geraldine Fitzgerald

The role of nutrition in the management of multiple sclerosis (MS) is often neglected despite evidence implicating nutritional factors in the aetiology of the disease (see Chapter 2). In addition, studies of the food intake of people with MS have been shown to be low in energy, zinc, copper, folate, calcium and B vitamins (Witschi *et al.*, 1970; Crawford and Stevens, 1981; Harding and Crawford, 1981; Hewson *et al.*, 1984). The provision of nutritional advice to people with a chronic disease such as MS is likely to prevent nutrient deficiencies occurring. It would seem sensible to suggest an increase in the nutrients which are involved in the support and maintenance of the central nervous system (CNS).

However, only a small proportion of people with MS appear to receive qualified nutritional advice following diagnosis. This was observed in a survey where 390 people, on entry to a nutrition and exercise programme, were asked if they had altered their diets as a result of having MS. Of the sample, 241 (61%) claimed to have made changes to their diet, but only 11% of them had received dietary advice from their doctors (Simpson and Hewson, 1985).

From the survey it would appear that some people with MS want to make changes to their diets but professional advice is not generally offered. The reasons why nutritional advice is not routinely available following diagnosis are not clear. A possible reason could be the number of different dietary therapies which are advocated in the treatment of MS. Some of these diets are based on scientific studies and trials while others rely on anecdotal evidence. Often the latter regimens offer the hope or expectation of a cure. Due to this, and the unproven evidence of some of the diets, it could be speculated that all diets are treated with caution or thought of as cranky or unhelpful by some of the professionals who work with MS. To dismiss nutrition in this way disregards the fact that some patients want to try to change their diet, and the role nutrition has in maintaining the general health of an individual. This chapter therefore discusses the available evidence on nutrition and its role in the management of MS.

EVIDENCE FOR A LOW FAT DIET RICH IN ESSENTIAL FATTY ACIDS

The majority of the research to date has been concerned with the fat content of the diet. Epidemiological studies have shown correlations between the incidence of MS and the amount of animal fat in the diet (Swank, 1950; Sinclair, 1956; Allison, 1963; Bernsohn and Stephanides, 1967; Agranoff and Goldberg, 1974; Dick 1976). Analysis of blood plasma and cell membranes of MS patients have shown low levels of the essential fatty acid (EFA), linoleic acid (Baker, Thompson and Zilkha, 1964; Thompson, 1966; Sanders *et al.*, 1968; Gul *et al.*, 1970; Neu, 1983; Cherayil, 1984). Abnormalities in the fatty acid composition of brain tissue in MS have also been reported (Thompson, 1975). Supplementation with linoleic acid in the form of sunflower oil, or as a spread, was studied in three double blind trials. Data from the three trials were analysed separately and then jointly (Millar *et al.*, 1973; Bates *et al.*, 1978; Paty *et al.*, 1978; Dworkin *et al.*, 1984). The results of the combined data looking at acute relapsing patients only, suggested a reduction in the number and severity of relapses and in the rate of deterioration in the treated group. This was most marked in those patients with minimal disability and duration of disease (Dworkin *et al.*, 1984). The results of a study investigating the effect of a low fat diet over 20 years have been published by Swank (1970) who claimed a reduction in the relapse rate and disability, was well as a reduction in the death rate.

THE IMPORTANCE OF THE EFAs IN RELATION TO MS

Essential fatty acids (EFA) are so called because they cannot be manufactured in the body, and therefore need to be obtained from food. There are two chains of EFAs, n-6 and n-3. The parent fatty acids are linoleic and alpha linolenic respectively. In the body the fatty acids are converted into long chain fatty acids, arachidonic, eicosapentaenoic and docosahexaenoic (see Figure 8.1), which are incorporated into cell membranes. Sixty percent of the solid matter

Figure 8.1 Schematic diagram showing the conversion of parent fatty acids into long-chain derivatives. Reproduced with permission from Action and Research for Multiple Sclerosis (ARMS).

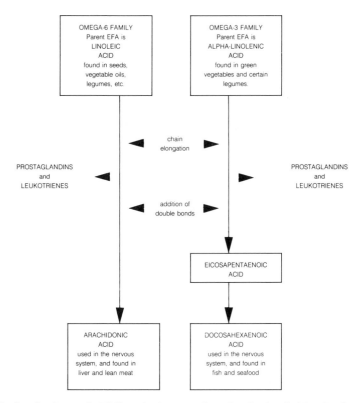

of the brain and 70% of the myelin sheath is lipid. Studies investigating the EFA component of the brain have found that the long chain derivatives of the parent fatty acids form the majority of EFAs (Crawford *et al.*, 1976).

The conversion of the parent fatty acids to their long chain derivatives is slow and it is the initial reaction which is thought to be rate limiting (Crawford *et al.*, 1979). Research investigating the conversion of linoleic and alpha linolenic fatty acids into the long chain derivatives has shown it requires 30 molecules of linoleic acid to yield one molecule of arachidonic acid, and 10 molecules of alpha linolenic to give one molecule of docosahexaenoic acid. It has also been found that preformed long chain derivatives are incorporated into the CNS many times faster than the parent fatty acids (Houtomuller, 1975).

The long chain derivatives of the fatty acids produce precursors of prostaglandins as well as forming part of cell membranes. There are implications for prostaglandin synthesis in MS as they have a role in vascular activity and the immune system. It has been suggested that autoimmune mechanisms play a part in the disease process and that via the formation of prostaglandins the polyunsaturated fats may be immunosuppressive (Gurr, 1983). Increased stickiness of platelets, decreased linoleic acid in lymphocytes and vascular disturbances in MS have been found (Wright, Thompson and Zilkha, 1965; Srivastava *et al.*, 1975; Tsang *et al.*, 1976). In contrast to this one of the prostaglandins formed from arachidonic acid is a precursor of prostacyclin, which prevents platelet adhesion. Increasing the intake of EFA may therefore have a preventative effect in the development of the above abnormalities.

THE EFA DIET

The EFA diet was proposed by Crawford *et al.* (1979), and contains sources of both families of EFAs, i.e. the parent fatty acids of linoleic and linolenic and their long chain derivatives, arachidonic acid, decosahexaenoic and eicosapentaenoic fatty acids. The latter are important due to the low conversion rate of the parent fatty acids in the body. The diet, while rich in EFAs, is low in saturated fat. An increase in polyunsaturates in the diet means there is likely to be an increased need for the nutrients which are involved in the conversion and protection of the fatty acids in the body. Examples of accessory nutrients are vitamins E and C which act as anti-oxidants and protect the polyunsaturates from oxidation in the body. Zinc, copper, and iron are involved in the synthesis of the long chain derivatives, as are the B vitamins. As a result of the probable increased need of such nutrients, levels above the recommended daily allowances set by the DHSS are advised as part of the EFA diet. The increased recommended intakes are based on those which could be achieved if an individual were following all the guidelines of the diet. Table 8.1 shows the target levels set by ARMS in 1980. The EFA diet revolves around three main areas of advice:

1. Increasing the sources of the EFAs in the diet;
2. decreasing the sources of saturated fats;
3. increasing nutrient dense foods to meet the ARMS targets and

Table 8.1 Target levels of nutrients. Reproduced with permission from John Libbey and Company Ltd.

Nutrient		British	ARMS target
Calories	M	2510	2000
	F	2150	1800
Fibre (g)		COMA/NACNE 30 g	30
Calcium (mg)	M	500	800
	F	500	800
Iron (mg)	M	10	16
	F	12	16
Copper (mg)		Average intake 1-3 mg/day	4
Zinc (mg)	M	Average intake 9-12 mg/day	12
	F		12
Retinol (μg)	M	750	Not > 6000
	F	750	Not > 6000
Vitamin D (μg)	M	Up to 10 μg	Up to 15 μg
	F	Up to 10 μg	Up to 15 μg
Thiamin (mg)	M	1.0	1.7
	F	0.9	1.5
Riboflavin (mg)	M	1.6	3.3
	F	1.3	3.0
Nicotinic acid (mg)	M	18	25
	F	15	23
Vitamin C (mg)	M	30	120
	F	30	120
Vitamin E (mg)	M	Average intake 5-10 mg/day	12
	F		12
Vitamin B$_{12}$ (μg)	M	3.4 μg	30
	F	3.4 μg	30
Folic acid total (μg)	M	300	350
	F	300	350
Vitamin B$_6$ (mg)	M	Average intake 1.5-2 mg/day	2.0
	F		2.0

the NACNE (1983) and COMA (DHSS, 1984) recommendations for general health.

Increasing the sources of the EFAs

Linoleic acid is found in polyunsaturated margarines and oils. Suitable margarines include sunflower, safflower and soya. For a margarine or oil to be acceptable they should be labelled 'high in polyunsaturates'. Oils that are suitable include sunflower, safflower, sesame seed, cotton seed, corn, soya, rapeseed, grapeseed and walnut. The majority of these oils are readily available from supermarkets. They contain high amounts of linoleic acid; some are higher than others but as they are all rich sources it is a question of personal taste which oil people prefer to use. Cold pressed oils are often advocated by purists, but the amounts of linoleic acid in the supermarket brands are sufficiently high for it not to be necessary to buy the more expensive cold pressed. Blends of vegetable oils should not be used as hydrogenation takes place and the oils do not contain sufficient polyunsaturates.

It is important to store oils in a cool place. Frying with polyunsaturated oils is best kept to a minimum, as heating causes hydrogenation, and as a result the oils become more saturated. Deep fat frying is discouraged, and the oil should only ever be used once, and not kept.

Linoleic acid is also found in nuts, pulses, seeds, legumes and beans, so these should be included regularly in the diet. Some people may be unaware of how to prepare beans and pulses, so recommending a good cookery book or providing a recipe leaflet can be helpful. Large amounts of nuts should not be eaten, as they are very high in fat, both saturated and polyunsaturated. Coconut is best avoided completely as it is very high in saturated fats. It is advised that peanuts should be kept to a minimum as some evidence suggests that they may be atherogenic.

The long chain derivative of linoleic acid is arachidonic acid. This is found in offal and lean meats. Liver is a rich source of arachidonic acid as well as many other nutrients, including the B vitamins, vitamin A, iron and zinc. Up to, but no more than, half a pound of liver should be eaten weekly as otherwise the vitamin A content of the diet is too high. Vitamin A is toxic in large amounts over long periods of time.

Liver tends to be one of the foods that many people have an aversion to, but its importance should be stressed. Without liver it is much more difficult for the nutritional targets for folic acid, zinc and B6 to be met. The reason why liver is so disliked is not always obvious. Some people find that it has too strong a taste, in which case they may prefer to try chicken liver which is milder than other kinds. The taste can be disguised and having recipe leaflets available can be helpful.

Other types of offal such as heart and kidneys are also recommended. Lean meats and poultry can be eaten, but all visible fat should be trimmed before cooking, and the skin from poultry removed. Game meats and birds such as rabbit, venison and partridges are very low in saturated fats and high in arachidonic acid. They are also becoming increasingly available from supermarkets.

The EFA alpha linolenic acid is found in green vegetables, beans, legumes and linseeds. It is advised that a large portion of green leafy vegetables such as cabbage, broccoli, spinach and spring greens should be eaten daily. Fresh or frozen vegetables are suitable, but tinned vegetables contain very little nutrients and should be avoided. There is a loss of nutrients during the cooking of vegetables so it is important not to over-cook them and to have a source of raw vegetables daily in the form of a salad. Linseeds are commercially available as 'Linusit Gold', from most health food shops. They are tiny golden seeds, and rich sources of the alpha linolenic acid. It is recommended that a dessertspoonful a day is eaten, sprinkled over salads, breakfast cereals, in casseroles or yoghurt. It also has a laxative effect, and if someone is suffering from constipation increasing the amounts of linseeds in the diet can relieve this.

The long chain derivatives of alpha linolenic are found in fish and seafood. It is advised that fish or seafood should be eaten three or four times a week and this should include an oily fish such as mackerel, herring, tuna, salmon and trout. Fresh fish or seafood is the best source, but if it is unavailable then frozen or tinned fish are acceptable. Tinned fish should ideally be in brine, but if in oil, it should be drained off before eating.

Decreasing the saturated fats

The sources of saturated fat fall into three main categories: dairy products, meat products and confectionery.

Dairy products

Butter is very high in saturated fat and is replaced in the EFA diet by polyunsaturated margarines. Cooking fats such as lard are replaced by the polyunsaturated oils. Milk should be skimmed. Many people find this too watery at first, but it would appear that this is something they become used to in a very short space of time, so much so that full fat milk then tastes too rich. Cream and anything containing cream should not be eaten. Cream can be replaced by natural yoghurt in cooking or on puddings and sweets. For special occasions greek yoghurt, which has 10% fat, can be used and although higher in fat than the natural yoghurt it is still much lower than cream. Full fat cheeses, such as cheddar or stilton, are to be avoided. Cheeses such as brie, edam or camembert are medium fat cheeses, but the amount eaten on a weekly basis should still be kept low. Cottage cheese, curd cheese, and fromage frais are all low fat and can be eaten freely. It is recommended that no more than three or four eggs should be eaten in a week. This is because yolks of eggs contain fat, and also eggs are high in cholesterol, which for general health it is advised to keep to a minimum.

Meat products

Fatty cuts of meat and meat product are high in saturated fat. Only lean cuts of meat should be eaten. Sausages, meat pies, shop bought pâtés and processed meats such as salami or garlic sausage should be avoided.

Confectionery

Shop-bought cakes, biscuits, pastries, some confectionery and snacks are high in fat. Pastry, cakes and biscuits made with wholemeal flour and a polyunsaturated margarine are an alternative. Chocolate and crisps are high in fat and should be replaced with low fat snacks such as dried fruit, sunflower seeds, fresh fruit or nuts.

Increasing nutrient dense foods

Unrefined foods are higher in nutrients than processed food. It is therefore recommended that wholemeal bread, cereals, pasta and brown rice are used in preference to the white variety. Sugar should be avoided, but if baking then an unrefined sugar such as muscovado or demerara can be used. Fresh fruit and fruit juices should be included on a daily basis, as they are rich in nutrients such as fibre, vitamin C and folic acid.

The EFA diet is summarized in Table 8.2.

The EFA diet study

The EFA diet was proposed so that people with MS could receive sound nutritional advice and, as discussed earlier, ensuring general health is one of the aims. The diet was also proposed as a result of previous research which suggested that increasing the EFA content of the diet had a therapeutic effect in MS, as was shown in the

Table 8.2 Summary of the diet rich in essential fatty acids. Reproduced with permission from Action and Research for Multiple Sclerosis (ARMS).

1. Use a polyunsaturated margarine and oils.
2. Eat at least three helpings of fish each week.
3. Eat ½lb liver each week.
4. Eat a large helping of dark green vegetables daily.
5. Eat some raw vegetables daily, as a salad, with French dressing.
6. Eat some linseeds or 'Linusit Gold' daily.
7. Eat some fresh fruit daily.
8. Try to eat as much fresh food as possible in preference to processed food.
9. Choose lean cuts of meat, and trim all fat away from meat before cooking.
10. Try to avoid hard animal fats like butter, lard, suet, dripping, and fatty foods such as cream, hard cheese, etc.
11. Try to eat wholegrain cereals and wholemeal bread rather than refined cereals.
12. Try to cut down on sugar and foods containing sugar.

sunflower oil trials (see above). The EFA diet is a total nutritional approach. The levels of linoleic acid in the diet are comparable to those in the sunflower trials, and the other EFAs are increased. Adequate intakes of vitamins, minerals, trace elements and fibre are ensured as part of the dietary advice.

As part of a disease management study, 83 patients with clinically defined MS were advised on a low saturated fat, high polyunsaturated fat diet. The average length of time in the study was 39 months (range 2–5 years). Compliance with the diet was monitored by analysis of 7-day weighed intakes using a nutrient scoring system at 6-monthly intervals and blood lipid analysis.

Subjects at differing levels of compliance were compared using the Kurtzke expanded disability status scale. Patients with a low level of compliance were found to have significantly deteriorated ($P < 0.022$) whilst those with a high level of compliance had not changed significantly throughout the study.

The changes in the fat content of the diet were consistent with those found in the blood plasma fatty acids. Correlations were found between the dietary linoleic acid and plasma choline phosphoglyceride (PC) linoleic acid. Correlations between the dietary long-chain n-3 fatty acids and the blood plasma PC eicosapentaenoic were found. These results reflect the dietary advice being followed and the emphasis of the diet that both chains of fatty acids should be included (Fitzgerald *et al.*, 1987).

111

Nutritional supplements

The taking of supplements by people with MS is very common, and many people take massive amounts of supplements generally based on advice from self-help type books. With the exception of supplementation with linoleic acid, there is no scientific evidence to suggest that supplements should be taken. It has previously been discussed that the amounts of linoleic used in the sunflower trials are available if a polyunsaturated oil and margarine are used rather than saturated fats. When the EFA diet is being followed closely there should be no need to take supplements as all nutrient requirements would be met. However, in the case of some individuals there may be a need for supplementation, either due to food aversions or poor appetite. Many people may still prefer to take a supplement, even though they have been advised that it is unnecessary. This may act as an 'insurance policy' or they may feel that it is something that they can do for themselves. In such a situation they should be advised to take a wide based multivitamin and mineral rather than a range of different tablets.

The most commonly taken supplement tends to be Evening Primrose Oil (EPO). This is an oil containing mainly the fatty acids, linoleic acid and gamma linolenic acid (GLA). GLA is the next fatty acid after linoleic in the conversion process to the long chain fatty acids, and it is this fatty acid that is supposed to give the EPO its therapeutic qualities. However, the amount of the GLA is very small in comparison to the linoleic acid. The only trial carried out investigating the effect of EPO on MS did not show it to be of benefit, in contrast to the results of sunflower oil supplementation (Bates *et al.*, 1978). It is important to point out to people that if they use a polyunsaturated oil and margarine, sufficient linoleic acid is obtained and they need not supplement with EPO. Other oils containing higher amounts of GLA have appeared on the market in recent years, including borage oil and blackcurrant seed oil. Again there is no need to take such supplements if the polyunsaturated oils and margarines are being used as part of the diet. The effects of such high amounts of GLA on the cell membranes of people with MS are not known.

Fish oils are also often advocated in MS (Bates *et al.*, 1989), but unless someone has an aversion to oily fish and is unable to eat one such meal a week, there does not seem to be any benefit in taking fish oil supplements. Anyone taking fish oil supplements needs to be aware of the high amount of vitamin A they contain. Liver also contains large amounts of vitamin A, which is toxic in high enough quantities. For this reason if fish oils are advised they should be ones which do not contain vitamin A, such as MAXEPA.

OTHER DIETS IN MS

Diets to gain or lose weight

Many people with MS may become overweight either due to a decrease in mobility with the same eating patterns or as a result of depression. Overweight in MS carries all the inherent risks that occur in the general population but also aggravates mobility problems and fatigue. In addition, if a patient is overweight, to the extent that the carer is unable to lift or transfer easily, the carer is in danger of injury, especially to the back.

Overweight is therefore an important issue in MS, and should be tackled before the gain is too great. In the case of a weight gain due to decreased mobility, re-education of eating habits needs to take place, so that they become accustomed to eating less. When someone is overeating as a result of depression, it is advisable to recommend counselling or self-help groups for people with eating problems. Most people will lose weight on 1000 calorie diets but in the severely disabled calories may need to drop below this. When this is the case patients should be monitored closely and possibly supplements prescribed if necessary to ensure that all the nutrient targets are met.

Underweight can also be a problem in MS, as there is often a loss of appetite. In such cases the individual should be encouraged to eat larger portions, supplemented with Complan type drinks. It may be that they are heavy smokers which will depress the appetite and the cessation of smoking should be strongly encouraged. Smoking should be discouraged in all MS patients. If the patient is anorexic then referral to a counsellor or psychotherapist is advocated. Eating, swallowing and chewing problems can all result in weight loss. Speech therapists can advise both the patient and dietitian on the best methods to overcome these problems and to prevent weight loss.

Gluten-free diets

Studies have indicated that the incidence of MS correlates with the areas of the world where wheat and rye are the prevalent cereals cultivated (Shatin, 1964). Abnormalities in the jejunal mucosa have also been found in some patients with MS (Lange and Shiner, 1976; Gupta *et al.*, 1977). These studies have led to the speculation of the involvement of gluten in the aetiology of MS, and that therefore the avoidance of gluten would have a therapeutic role in the treatment of MS.

The most publicized information on gluten-free diets is the anecdotal evidence of Rita Greer (1982) and Roger McDougall (1989). Both devised diets which are generally thought of as gluten-free. Both are more complicated. The Roger McDougall diet is gluten-free, low fat, contains no refined sugar and large doses of multi-vitamins are taken. He claims that by developing such a diet over a period of four years, he recovered to the extent of being able to walk again. Rita Greer developed a gluten-free, dairy products-free, sugar-free diet which also contains no meat or oily fish. This was developed for her husband who had MS. Again she claims that over a period of several years he recovered from being in a wheelchair to being able to walk. Both these accounts are obviously highly emotive, and it is easy to understand why someone with MS would be keen to try such diets.

However, studies investigating the therapeutic effect of a gluten-free diet have been unable to demonstrate any clinical benefits (Liversedge, 1977; Hewson, 1984). In Liversedge's study, 40 patients were followed over two years on a gluten-free diet. Of the 37 who completed the trial the relapse rate was no better than average and the disability scores worsened as expected for untreated groups. In the latter study it was shown that people on a gluten-free diet tended to have lower calorie intakes, were likely to be taking large amounts of unnecessary supplements, mainly of B vitamins. Out of 22 patients, six were consuming less than 15g fibre per day, which is less than half the NACNE recommendations. Overall it would appear that there is insufficient evidence to recommend a gluten-free diet to patients with MS.

The Swank low fat diet

The Swank low fat diet (Swank and Duggan, 1987) differs from the EFA diet in that it gives precise amounts of the fats and oils which are to be consumed on a daily basis. The amount of saturated fat per day should not exceed 15g and the polyunsaturates contained in the diet should be between 20g and 50g. No red meat can be eaten in the first year of following the diet. Professor Swank also prescribes cod-liver oil supplements and a multivitamin and mineral tablet. The results of a 20 year study of MS patients following the diet has been published (Swank, 1970). He claims that by following the diet there is a decrease in the number of relapses, and a marked slowing down of the disease process. His work has been criticized as it is not a double-blind trial, and he also uses a different neurological scale. Nonetheless, when viewed in the light of the sunflower oil trials and the results of the EFA study, it forms part of the growing amount of data indicating the therapeutic aspects of a low saturated fat and EFA rich diet.

Vegans and vegetarians

Vegetarians and vegans cannot be said to follow an EFA diet due to the diet's emphasis on the long chain fatty acids and their sources. They can, however, follow a low fat diet that is rich in the parent fatty acids. It has not been established whether such a diet would be as therapeutic as a diet containing all sources of EFAs. It is possible to meet the targets for all the other nutrients on a vegetarian or vegan diet, but may require greater attention being paid to the food eaten. Supplements of B12 are likely to be needed.

The reason why someone is vegetarian or vegan needs to be discussed. In some cases it may be that the main reason is as a therapeutic diet for MS, in which case they may consider including fish and liver in their diet. If it is for moral or ethical reasons then the advice is to have a low fat vegetarian diet, and to avoid the full fat dairy products.

Allergy diets

There is a growing amount of interest in the role of allergies in MS. At present there is no evidence which links the two together. Some of the claims made for the effects of food allergies are very dramatic and this has led to many people visiting clinical ecologists or sending blood and hair samples away to be analysed. The methods used for diagnosing allergies vary, but it would appear that methods such as applied kinesiology and hair analysis are very difficult to replicate (Lessof, 1986).

The most thorough way to test for allergies is by an elimination diet, although this is time consuming and should only be done under the strict supervision of a dietitian.

GUIDELINES TO DIETITIANS AND NUTRITIONISTS

From the available evidence the EFA diet is the one which is the most comprehensive from both a general health and therapeutic aspect. It combines the low fat approach of Swank with the linoleic acid effect of the sunflower oil trials. As discussed above, there is also an increase in the long chain fatty acids and the parent fatty acid of the n-3 family. Nutrient dense foods are advised to increase the intake of vitamins, minerals, trace elements and fibre. It is also suitable for the whole family and should not involve the preparation of separate meals for the person with MS. The EFA diet is therefore felt by the author to be the most suitable to advise on. The following guidelines are therefore based on the EFA diet.

In the ideal situation the dietitian would see the person with MS soon after diagnosis. This tends not to be the case, and allows for many misconceptions to arise over and above personal beliefs about food. Whenever the first advice session takes place it is important for the diet to be explained clearly and concisely.

The advice session can be split into three main sections:

1. Introducing the idea of the diet, explaining the scientific background and history of the diet. The level of detail will depend very much on the individual patient as to how much they feel they want to know.
2. Explaining the different types of fat, and the sources of poly-unsaturated and saturated fats. Explaining what the EFA diet consists of, foods to include and foods to avoid. Introducing the concept of nutrient dense food and why they are important.
3. Taking a diet history to assess the individual's diet and explain-ing how adaptations can be made. The family situation needs to be considered and advice offered to other family members if necessary, particularly if the person with MS is not doing the shopping and cooking.

The session should be ended by offering advice on supplements, answering queries about other diets in MS. Space should be given throughout the consultation to allow the individual to ask questions.

A diet booklet and recipe sheets should be provided for the individual to take away with them.

Such a consultation will take a long time and a great deal of information is imparted. Fifty percent of information is said to be forgotten within ten minutes of receiving it, and people with MS may have memory problems so follow-up sessions are very important. It is also unrealistic to expect some people to change their diet as a result of one session as it has taken them a lifetime to develop their eating habits.

Finding out which changes to their diet have been made, and providing positive feed-back should be part of the follow-up sessions. If certain parts of the diet are not being followed this needs to be discussed and the reasons explored. It may be due to food aversions, particularly in the case of, for example, liver and other offal. Or it may be that people need to get used to some changes in their way of eating before they can accommodate further adaptations to the way they eat.

Some people may not make changes to their diets, or reverse changes that were previously made. This will only become apparent if follow-up assessments are carried out regularly. Expectations of the diet and how it may affect the course of MS may be involved. During the initial session the patient's expectations of the diet should be discussed, but these may remain unrealistic. Even if someone is following the diet very closely their MS is still likely to get worse and in some cases the deterioration will be quite marked. Some people with rapid deterioration may feel there is no point in continuing with a diet under such circumstances. The effect of the EFA diet would appear to be preventative. Subjectively some people may feel better, but it will not cause a reversal of the damage done to the nervous system by the MS. Reinforcing the idea of the possible preventative effect may not be enough for some people if they had expected a cure. However, talking about these expectations can be helpful and in some cases clarifying the difficulties and unreality can be enough to re-motivate them into adhering to the diet more closely.

The practical difficulties of following the diet for some people, particularly for those who may be more disabled and living alone, need to be recognized. Some problems can be solved by making use of the services of specialists such as occupational therapists, speech therapists and continence advisers.

The dietitian or nutritionist has to be clear about her own expectations and not feel undermined or get sucked into despair.

Acknowledging the limitations of the diet and her own role is essential. She can only be responsible for providing sound dietary advice in what may be a changing situation, and for supporting the individual and be aware of the value of such a role.

It also has to be recognized that diet is one of many therapies available and that it will probably be only part of a self-help regimen that the person with MS is carrying out. The extent to which the individual feels able to use the dietary advice may be altered by their commitment to other therapies. There is only so much a person can take on board at any one time, and some people with MS may choose to give another therapy, such as counselling or physiotherapy, a higher profile for a while before they come back to following the diet.

The person with MS must also be aware of how to adapt the diet to fit in with their life style and family life. It is important to ensure that changes are made gradually and smoothly to minimize disruption. The dietitian should be aware of how disruptive these changes can be to families.

SUMMARY AND CONCLUSIONS

Nutrition has an important role in the management of MS. The role is three-fold: to provide advice on the general health aspects of diet, to provide nutritional education and to provide advice about the therapeutic role of diet in MS. The EFA diet is such that all the family can follow it and benefit. Therefore the person with MS need not follow a separate diet from the rest of the family.

Referrals to a dietitian should be sought as soon as possible and with sound dietetic support the EFA diet can be followed by people with all levels of disability. The evidence so far is encouraging and research is continuing and developing.

REFERENCES

Agranoff, B. and Goldberg, D. (1974) Diet and the geographical distribution of multiple sclerosis. *Lancet,* **ii**, 1061–6.

Allison, R. (1963) Some neurological aspects of medical geography. *Proceedings of the Royal Society of Medicine,* **56**, 71–6.

Baker, R., Thompson, R. and Zilkha, K. (1964) Serum fatty acids and multiple sclerosis. *Journal of Neurology, Neurosurgery and Psychiatry,* **27**, 408–14.

Bates, D., Fawcett, P.R.W., Shaw, D.A. *et al.* (1978) Polyunsaturated fatty acids in the treatment of acute remitting multiple sclerosis. *British Medical Journal,* **2**, 1390–1.

Bates, D., Belin, J., Cartlidge, N.E.F. *et al.* (1989) A double-blind controlled trial of long chain n-3 polyunsaturated fatty acids in the treatment of multiple sclerosis. *Journal of Neurology, Neurosurgery and Psychiatry,* **52**, 18–22.

Bernsohn, J. and Stephanides, L.M. (1967) Aetiology of multiple sclerosis. *Nature* (London), **215**, 821.

Cherayil, G.D. (1984) Sialic acid and fatty acid concentrations in lymphocytes, red blood cells, and plasma from patients with multiple sclerosis. *Journal of Neurological Sciences,* **63**, 1–10.

Crawford, M.A., Hassam, A., Williams, G. *et al.* (1976) Essential fatty acids and foetal brain growth. *Lancet,* **i**, 452.

Crawford, M.A., Budowski, P. and Hassam, A.G. (1979) Dietary management in multiple sclerosis. *Proceedings of the Nutrition Society,* **38**, 373–89.

Crawford, M.A. and Stevens, P. (1981) A study on essential fatty acids and multiple sclerosis. *Progress in Lipid Research,* **20**, 255–7.

DHSS (1984) Diet and cardiovascular disease. Committee on Medical Aspects (COMA) of Food Policy, Report on Health and Social Subjects No.28. HMSO, London.

Dick, G. (1976) The aetiology of multiple sclerosis. *Proceedings of the Royal Society of Medicine,* **69**, 611–16.

Dworkin, R.H., Bates, D., Millar, J.H.D. *et al.* (1984) Linoleic acid and multiple sclerosis: a re-analysis of three double blind trials. *Neurology,* **34**, 1441–5.

Fitzgerald, G.E., Simpson, K.E., Harbige, L.S. *et al.* (1987) The effect of nutritional counselling on dietary compliance and disease course in multiple sclerosis patients over three years, in *Multiple Sclerosis: Immunological, Diagnostic and Therapeutic Aspects,* Current problems in Neurology No.3. Chap.26, (eds F. Clifford Rose and R. Jones). John Libbey Pubs.Co., London and Paris, pp. 189–99.

Greer, R. (1982) *Diets to Help Multiple Sclerosis.* Thorsons, Northants.

Gul, S., Smith, A.D., Thompson, R.H.S. *et al.* (1970) Fatty acid composition of phospholipids from platelets and erythrocytes in multiple sclerosis. *Journal of Neurology, Neurosurgery and Psychiatry,* **33**, 506–10.

Gupta, J., Ingengno, A., Cook, A. *et al.* (1977) Multiple sclerosis and malabsorption. *American Journal of Gastroenterology,* **68**, 560.

Gurr, M.I. (1983) The role of lipids in the regulation of the immune system. *Progress in Lipid Research,* **22**, 257–87.

Harding, J. and Crawford, M.A. (1981) The role of diet in multiple sclerosis. *Applied Nutrition,* **1** (BDA Study Conference), 20–3.

Hewson, D.C. (1984) Is there a role for gluten-free diets in multiple sclerosis? *Human Nutrition: Applied Nutrition,* **38A**, 417–20.

Hewson, D.C., Phillips, M.A., Simpson, K.E. *et al.* (1984) Food intake in multiple sclerosis. *Human Nutrition: Applied Nutrition,* **30A**, 355–67.

Houtomuller, U.M.T. (1975) Specific biological effects of polyunsaturated fatty acids, in *The Role of Fats in Human Nutrition,* (ed. A.J. Vergroessen). Academic Press, London, pp. 331–51.

119

Lange, L.S. and Shiner, H. (1976) Small bowel abnormalities in multiple sclerosis. *Lancet*, **ii**, 1319–22.

Lessof, M.H. (1986) Allergy and its mechanisms. *British Medical Journal*, **292**, 385–7.

Liversedge, L.A. (1977) Treatment and management of multiple sclerosis. *British Medical Bulletin*, **33**, 78–83.

McDougall, R. (1989) *My Fight Against Multiple Sclerosis*. Regenics Pubn., Chorley, Lancs.

Millar, J.H.D., Zilkha, K.S., Langman, M.J.S. *et al.* (1973) Double blind trial of linoleate supplementation of the diet in multiple sclerosis. *British Medical Journal*, **1**, 765–8.

NACNE (1983) A discussion paper on proposals for nutritional guidelines for health education in Britain. The National Advisory Committee on Nutrition: Education Working Party chaired by Prof. W.P.T. James. Health Education Council Publication, London.

Neu, I.S. (1983) Essential fatty acids in the serum and cerebrospinal fluid of multiple sclerosis patients. *Acta Neurologica Scandinavica*, **67**, 151–63.

Paty, D.W., Cousin, H.K., Read, S. *et al.* (1978) Linoleic acid in multiple sclerosis: failure to show any therapeutic benefit. *Acta Neurologica Scandinavica*, **58**, 53–8.

Sanders, H., Thompson, R.H.S., Wright, H.P. *et al.* (1968) Further studies on platelet adhesiveness and serum cholesteryl linoleate levels in multiple sclerosis. *Journal of Neurology, Neurosurgery and Psychiatry*, **31**, 321–5.

Shatin, R. (1964) Multiple sclerosis and geography: new interpretation of epidemiological observations. *Neurology (Minneap.)*, **14**, 338.

Simpson, K.E. and Hewson, D. (1985) Food intake in multiple sclerosis. *Proceedings of the 2nd International Congress on EFAs, PGs and Leukotrienes*. The Zoological Society of London, March.

Sinclair, H. (1956) Deficiency of essential fatty acids and atherosclerosis. *Lancet*, **i**, 381.

Srivastava, K.C., Foc, T. and Clausen, J. (1975) The synthesis of prostaglandins in platelets from patients with multiple sclerosis. *Acta Neurologica Scandinavica*, **51**, 193–9.

Swank, R.L. (1950) Multiple sclerosis: a correlation of its incidence with dietary fat. *American Journal of Medical Science*, **220**, 441–50.

Swank, R.L. (1970) Multiple sclerosis: 20 years on a low-fat diet. *Archives of Neurology*, **23**, 460–74.

Swank, R.L. and Duggan, B.B. (1987) *The Multiple Sclerosis Diet Book: A low fat diet for the treatment of MS*. Doubleday and Co.Inc., New York.

Thompson, R.H.S. (1966) A biochemical approach to the problem of multiple sclerosis. *Proceedings of the Royal Society of Medicine*, **59**, 269–76.

Thompson, R.H.S. (1975) Unsaturated fatty acids in multiple sclerosis, in *Multiple Sclerosis Research* (eds A.N. Davison, J.H. Humphry, A.L. Liversedge *et al.*) USA: Elsevier, North Holland, pp. 184–93.

Tsang, N., Smith, A., Weyman, C. *et al.* (1976) Immunosuppression by fatty acids. *Lancet*, **ii**, 254.

Wright, H.P., Thompson, R.H.S. and Zilkha, K.J. (1965) Platelet adhesiveness in multiple sclerosis. *Lancet*, **ii**, 1109–10.

Witschi, J.C., Littell, A.S., Houser, H.B. *et al.* (1970) Dietary intake of non-hospitalized persons with multiple sclerosis. *Journal of American Dietetic Association*, **56**, 203–11.

9

Nursing

Kay Smithers

The person who has multiple sclerosis (MS) presents nursing with a series of challenges. This chapter explores the ways nursing can meet these in a variety of settings, both hospital and community based. In considering the complexities and unpredictable nature of the disease, the available strategies of nursing and their application, as well as some common problems and the research-based knowledge available to help overcome them, will be discussed. References are provided that will allow the reader to begin to explore these in more depth. In this chapter the term 'nurse' will refer to any nurse, health visitor or midwife in any speciality.

MS is a chronic, unpredictable and varied disease process which has a unique effect on each individual. It is therefore not possible to offer a blueprint of nursing care. The development of patient-centred, systematic problem solving as an approach to nursing (the Nursing Process), the examination of nursing philosophy through nursing models, and the rapid increase in nursing related research, allow nurses to plan appropriate care to help meet the challenges presented.

There are a variety of books available that discuss MS and these can provide the nurse with valuable insight into living with the disease (Burnfield, 1985; Graham, 1987; Forsythe, 1988; Lechtenberg, 1988). Nursing is a diverse activity occurring in any setting, which involves meeting the health needs of any patient within the context of their family and support system. The nurse will need to consider the individual with MS in the context of either the 'patient' or the 'carer'. The cause of contact may not be the MS itself, as those who have MS also experience the same patterns of health and illness as any one else, e.g. pregnancy, appendicitis, old age, etc. The carer of a patient may have MS, for example the wife of a heart attack victim, the mother of the new baby, the supportive daughter of the frail old lady, etc. In reality, the nurses most likely to have frequent contact with those who have MS will work on neurological and medical wards in district general hospitals, and in the community.

In order to discuss here what is meant by nursing care it is necessary to consider how nursing has been defined in relation to chronic illness. Many authors agree that the attitude of the nurse towards the concept of chronic illness is fundamental to the giving of appropriate care (Kratz, 1978; Davis, 1984). To date, researchers have found that nurses tend to have a negative and pessimistic attitude which in some cases has led to them withdrawing from the patient. Stockwell (1984), van Maanen (1981) and McClymont (1985) have identified the caring aspects of rehabilitative nursing (i.e. 'that which aims to restore the individual to his or her former state' (van Maanen, 1981)) to be split between self-care, and professional care. The main activities of the nurse are described as being educating, supporting, counselling and practical interventions. The latter may consist of doing things directly with the individual or referral to other agencies more suited to providing the required assistance. All these activities will be aimed at helping the individual achieve self-care and/or helping the community carers in their roles. The nurse should, where possible, work at the direction of the patient, whether helping to lift out of bed, planning the day's activities, or organizing outside help.

Price (1980) and Hanson (1987) amongst others have emphasized that nursing, especially when involved with the chronically ill, should not be focused solely on the patient but that all care should be based on the family unit or supporting group, and rehabilitative nursing follows this view. Similarly, many models require an assessment of self-care ability and support systems, and, without necessarily stating it, require family involvement. The supportive aspect of nursing care is vital but difficult to evaluate. People with MS have said that they would like to talk with someone who will just listen to their fears, hopes, worries and decisions. This person should ideally be from outside the support unit or family so that emotion can be 'off-loaded' without fear of hurting or offending, and without feeling guilty at 'sounding off' to hardworking spouses and friends. Community nurses are well placed for building up a long-term relationship that allows this to happen.

In the context of MS, the disease process is not an episode that will be over and done with, but is part of that person's way of life and always will be until such time as there is a cure. Life is to be lived either with MS, in spite of MS, or beside MS. Until quite

Figure 9.1 The nursing process

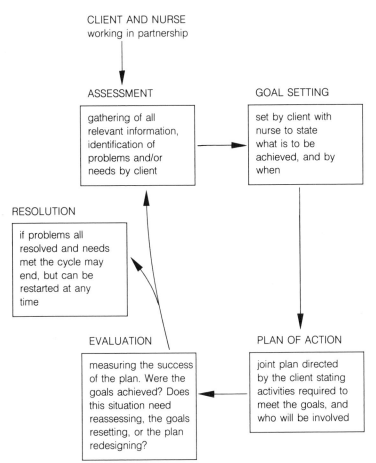

CLIENT AND NURSE
working in partnership

ASSESSMENT

gathering of all
relevant information,
identification of
problems and/or
needs by client

GOAL SETTING

set by client with
nurse to state
what is to be
achieved, and by
when

RESOLUTION

if problems all
resolved and needs
met the cycle may
end, but can be
restarted at any
time

EVALUATION

measuring the success
of the plan. Were the
goals achieved? Does
this situation need
reassessing, the goals
resetting, or the plan
redesigning?

PLAN OF ACTION

joint plan directed
by the client stating
activities required to
meet the goals, and
who will be involved

recently nursing textbooks acknowledged this in a rather gloomy and
fatalistic fashion. The truth is that most people with MS are trying
to get on with their lives and achieve their own goals as well as their
physical condition and its consequences will let them. Slater and
Yearwood (1980) claim that in the USA 80% of patients with MS
live a normal lifespan and 50% are still working ten years after
diagnosis. The authors consider that these figures could be improved
with appropriate rehabilitative care.

The Nursing Process provides a systematic framework for assessing situations and planning possible actions. This method of problem
solving can be used with any nursing model. Used for many years

in the USA, it has been formally adopted in the UK and is in various stages of implementation. The framework consists of several stages, all interlinked and interdependent. These are given various names but for the purpose of this discussion the sequence will be as indicated in Figure 9.1. As illustrated, these stages have a cyclical relationship and this is a helpful concept in meeting the needs of someone with a disease as variable and varying as MS. The cyclical pattern means that the patient's condition is constantly being reassessed and the care given evaluated as to its effectiveness. This allows for fluctuations in the MS and its effects, and consequent adjustments to the care planned. The application of a nursing model provides the philosophical background to the way in which the assessment and consequent planning of care is carried out. All models, be they based on activities of living (Roper, Logan and Tierney, 1980), the notion of self-care (Orem, 1980), or looking at the individual's adaptation to the situation (Roy, 1976), delineate the nurse–patient relationship as being patient-centred, and all nursing care as aimed at achieving the individual's potential, promoting health, minimizing difficulties, and preventing problems.

The assessment, or information gathering stage, is crucial, in that without it the subsequent stages are impossible to determine. However, nurses should only concentrate on the information that is needed to be able to plan care, and not invade personal privacy. The need for any information must be clearly explained. There are various skills involved in communication, which will be a vital component of any nurse–patient relationship. In the assessment stage the nurse needs to understand the individual's experience and point of view. Listening skills are therefore vital. Communication of information should be efficient between health care team members, although it is also important to respect the individual's right to confidentiality, and the nurse should check that the patient is happy for the information to be shared with other members of the team. The patient will also have identified and developed various strategies for living with MS and so will have some of the most important information that will determine the goals that are to be set and the care that must be planned. The patient also knows what sort of life he wants to lead therefore goal setting must be realistic and specific. Most models require that the patient is the goal setter, which meets the need expressed by many with MS to have control over their lives.

The nurse will meet the patient at various stages, starting probably at diagnosis. To become an 'accepted patient' and thus obtain help from a variety of agencies, financial benefits and access to most professional carers, one needs to have a recognizable condition that has been sanctioned by a member of the medical profession. With many illnesses this is easy enough. Some diseases, like MS, are notoriously difficult to diagnose in the initial stages, although current research may help remedy this. People with MS initially experience bizarre and usually transitory symptoms which only they can identify, and which are not visible to another person, although their effects may be, e.g. staggering, slurred speech. Many symptoms will go quickly and the individual will dismiss them, perhaps feeling that they can be explained by having 'overdone things'. Others will lead to a medical consultation. Some of the symptoms, such as numbness and fatigue, are easy to dismiss by both patient and doctor, especially when there seems to be no apparent pattern to their occurrence. Until a diagnosis is confirmed, people with MS express intense anxiety, often thinking that other people do not believe them, and they may start to think that they are 'going mad'. With the increase in the use of nurses in GP surgeries as an alternative port of call for those who consider that their problems may not require medical attention, the surgery or practice nurse may detect that a series of transitory problems is occurring and alert the GP. All professionals therefore need to keep detailed records.

It cannot be easy for the doctor to give the diagnosis, especially knowing that there is no definite treatment available to offer, but research has shown that people usually feel a sense of relief at being able to put a name to all that they have been going through (Gorman, Rudd and Ebers, 1984). Families are also known to cope with the situation more easily if given this information, but this must be with the individual's consent. The diagnosis will probably be followed by a quest for information starting in hospital, where many will be admitted for diagnosis, and continuing at home. The information required will obviously cover the disease itself and the possible effects that it may have on life style. But patients and their families will also want to know what they can do to improve their health, reduce the risk of long-term disability and lead a normal life. It is often the nurse who has the role of giving or reinforcing information. Details of the disease, health enhancing activities, help available, aids, support groups, agencies and benefits, could all be provided on information sheets to reinforce the verbal sessions. The information should be given when the patient and family are receptive and best able to remember what is said, and should be repeated as necessary. All information should be aimed at promoting self-care where possible (Levin, 1978). Patient education should constitute a large portion of the nurse's activity (Wilson-Barnett, 1983; Ewles and Simnett, 1985).

The individual's initial response and subsequent way of coping with and adapting to having MS will affect his attitudes and motivation in the areas discussed here. Many experience periods of denial, anger, depression, and finally acceptance, as if they are grieving for their lost health (Forsythe, 1988). This is discussed more fully elsewhere in this book.

The years following diagnosis will have an unspecified and unpredictable pattern. There may be long periods of remission, short attacks from which the individual rapidly recovers, a steady state or a rapid or steady decline in health functioning (Slater and Yearwood, 1980). The normal family concerns will be occurring simultaneously and the individual as spouse, parent or supporter of ageing parents, will be part of them. For this reason community nurses, along with other members of the primary health care team and social services, will be involved at various times to provide the support and back-up required. If a state of severe disability is reached, many people may be involved in the family situation, and the nurse should then act as team co-ordinator to reduce the number of intrusions into the family and ensure minimum disruption. Once contact is made with a patient who has MS, this should be reinforced at regular intervals, so that when a relapse does occur, or a difficulty arises, a working relationship between nurse and patient already exists.

Long and Phipps (1985, p.394) have derived a list of problems and unmet needs that most frequently occur in MS and which can be addressed by nurses. Other suggested care plans are discussed by Catanzaro (1980), McDonnell *et al.* (1980) and Ulrich, Canale and Wendell (1986). These have been categorized further for the purposes of this discussion and the combined result is shown in Figure 9.2. This gives a list of areas of concern that it is commonly agreed should be considered when assessing the patient and his or her situation. Any categorization of this kind is inevitably arbitrary, and many of the components of each group are interrelated to those in other groups. Key areas only will be discussed in this chapter.

PHYSICAL ACTIVITIES

Everyday activities, such as elimination, hygiene and grooming, mobility, feeding and sexual activity, will be considered.

Figure 9.2 Areas of concern to be considered when assessing the patient with multiple sclerosis.

PHYSICAL ACTIVITIES	PHYSICAL DISTURBANCES
mobility - reduced	pain
- impaired	
eating/drinking	loss of sensation
nutrition and fluid balance	loss of balance
cooking and shopping	loss of skin integrity
washing/dressing	fatigue
elimination - incontinence	visual disturbance
- constipation	speech difficulty
sexual activity	reactions to temperature
personal safety	
PSYCHOLOGICAL/EMOTIONAL	SOCIAL
lack of knowledge	isolation
need to communicate	need to maintain relationships
mood changes	employment
anxiety and fear	finance
frustration	carrying out normal roles
loss of concentration	- parent, partner, etc.
coping with chronic illness	control over one's life
depression	

Elimination

The controlled elimination of body wastes from the bladder and the bowel are something many people take for granted, except for the occasional bout of constipation or a holiday 'bug'. However, many women in the population are thought to have stress urinary incontinence following childbirth (Glew, 1986). With MS, incontinence (described by Boore (1980) as 'the passing of urine at the wrong time in the wrong place') is a worrying, embarrassing and depressing problem. Many feel ashamed that they have lost bladder control. Not everyone with MS will be incontinent, and if they are, it may be no more than a passing symptom. For some it may be that loss of sensation means that they are not sure when their bladder needs emptying. In this instance a regular routine of going to the toilet every two hours during the daytime will probably regain control. For others the difficulty to getting to the toilet and manipulating clothes fastenings may mean that 'accidents' happen. Again some kind of anticipatory routine, easier clothes fastenings, and the use of a walking aid may be enough. In fact, Thomas, Karran and Meade (1981) found that in a survey of 50 MS patients (of whom 43 had incontinence problems), 33 were helped by the introduction of services readily available. The identification of the problem is perhaps the most difficult aspect. The maintenance of continence or the living with incontinence without social embarrassment is of real importance to many people with MS. Apart from close family, it is often the nurse who is most likely to become aware of the problem. One of the most difficult aspects of incontinence is to talk about it and the individual may need to be presented with opportunities to do so on several occasions. The assessment of eliminative function will occur as part of many model-based assessments, and the need for a trusting relationship and comfortable interview technique cannot be over-emphasized. Norton (1986; pp. 55–7) outlines a useful assessment checklist. In addition to bowel and bladder habit it is concerned with such areas as mobility, psychological state, social network, environment and physical examination, and its use could clarify the approach to the problem that is most likely to succeed.

Many health authorities now have incontinence advisers (Smith, 1988) whose advice can be sought if appropriate and who may have input to in-service study days so that all staff can develop their skills in dealing with this problem. Liaison with other health professionals whose remit is covered more fully elsewhere in this book may also be required. For example, the physiotherapist can help with mobility, and the occupational therapist with equipment and, possibly, the fitting of a downstairs toilet. The medical staff may need to refer the client for urodynamic tests, in order to detect any malfunction in the way the bladder empties. Occasionally medical intervention may be required.

Incontinence is multi-factorial and one of the best ways of tackling it is prevention and education of the individual and carer to promote continence. The attitude adopted by the nurse should be positive and active. What can be done therefore to promote continence? A regular toilet routine has already been mentioned and will at least avoid most accidents during the day, as well as making it easier for the individual to get to the toilet and adopt the desired position to eliminate. If the pelvic floor muscles are weak, simple exercises may be taught for strengthening them, and the physiotherapist can help with these. Some people are tempted to reduce their fluid intake in the hope that they will be able to reduce the frequency with which they need to go to the toilet: this is dangerous in that it can lead to dehydration and may encourage urinary tract infections (UTI). Chronic infections of this kind can in turn lead to renal infection and possible failure, a not uncommon cause of death amongst people with MS. A UTI will also cause frequency and so the individual will end up having to go to the toilet more often than usual anyway. It may be possible to reduce the chances of nocturia by drinking more in the morning and early afternoon than in the evening, but the daily fluid intake must be satisfactory, i.e. at least a litre in 24 hours (Boore, Champion and Ferguson, 1987; p.833).

The importance of protection of the skin from excoriation and soreness is vital for comfort, well-being and to prevent infection. There are many products on the market aimed at skin care, from barrier creams to protective clothing, absorbent pads and waterproof sheets. The local health authority will be able to supply some of these, but they may not suit everybody's needs. Again the incontinence adviser or the local Aids for Living unit may be able to suggest alternatives. It is important that the nurse makes sure the individual knows what is available through these sources as many products are available commercially and the patient could incur unnecessary expense. Unfortunately there is little nursing research to identify which of these are most useful and the best way to use them, although the nursing press does occasionally report trials of such products, as do many publications aimed at the disabled. The fire danger of so-called 'inco' pads should be noted, especially if the client is a smoker with reduced manual dexterity. It is possible in some areas to make use of a laundry service, thereby reducing the workload of the individual or carer.

Also available, for men, are penile sheaths that drain into a collecting bag. These do not suit everyone as they require a degree of manual dexterity, and care must be taken to ensure that the individual is not allergic to rubber. Some patients may require catheterization, and much work has been done in recent years to commend the use of intermittent self-catheterization (CURN, 1982). This has been shown to have good results in terms of low infection rates but again relies on a degree of manual dexterity. Permanent catheterization should be the last choice because of the very high risk of infection and threat to the renal system that this would present. In some cases the risk of infection from urinary stasis, due to incomplete bladder emptying, outweighs this. There is much literature available regarding the prevention of infection in permanent catheters (Wilson and Roe, 1986).

The social effects of incontinence can be far-reaching. It is a miserable experience, and fear of embarrassment can lead to self-imposed isolation. Incontinence can also place a terrific burden on carers in terms of laundry, the effort of regularly helping someone to change soiled clothing and the cleaning of furniture and carpets. If the incontinence also includes that of the bowel, it is an even greater problem; however in MS constipation is more likely to occur than faecal incontinence (Matthews *et al.*, 1985). It is anticipated that through current research and by improvements in both resources and products, the individual will be able either to overcome the problem of incontinence or to live with it in such a way as to minimize its effects on other activities.

Mobility

The other activities mentioned in Figure 9.2 are encompassed in other parts of the book but a few points can be made. The mobility and manipulative skills, arm strength, etc., will affect the individual's ability to wash, dress, shop, cook, eat. Therefore a clear assessment of life style is important as is the referral to agencies, such as home-help, if required.

Sexual activity

Problems of sexual activity have been identified with MS (Matthews *et al.*, 1985) and suggestions of ways to help overcome these are discussed by Burnfield (1985), Graham (1987) and Lechtenberg (1988). SPOD (the Association to Aid Sexual and Personal Relationships of People with a Disability) have many useful publications, and some groups, e.g. ARMS, can provide supportive counselling. Sexual problems are the sort of problems that will only be aired once a trusting relationship has been established. Glower *et al.* (1986) have identified such problems in patients with neurological diseases. Of the men with MS in their sample 70% had sexual difficulties. Matthews *et al.* (1985) found that in men with MS the difficulty is likely to be erectile impotence, and in women loss of sensation, fatigue and reduced libido. Spasticity can be a problem for either sex, as can muscle weakness, making some positions difficult. Skilled counsellors will be needed to deal with the difficult problems, but the nurse will play an important role in identifying the problems, and acknowledging the sexuality of the individual. This will be linked to all aspects of their life and not just their sex life (Webb, 1985). As with all activities, sexual activity may need to be planned into the day's timetable. Although this takes away some spontaneity, it does mean that the couple have sufficient energy and time to enjoy the experience. At the time of diagnosis most people with MS are young adults and will therefore want to discuss family planning, fertility and child-care ability. There is no reason why, with the right support network, they should not go on to be as successful parents as anyone else. Research is currently under way to explore the experiences of mothers with MS (Smithers, 1988).

Physical disturbances

Many physical disturbances are transitory, but their effects are far-reaching. They also present symptoms that are generally invisible to others.

Some people (approximately 35%) experience pain in conjunction with their MS (Matthews, 1985), either as a primary symptom, for example trigeminal neuralgia, or as a secondary symptom, such as low back pain due to postural abnormality. There are a variety of methods dealing with pain and many of them do not involve drugs, e.g. position, warmth, massage, rest and transcutaneous electrical nerve stimulation.

A large number (73%) of MS patients experience sensory changes and optic nerve abnormalities (48%) (Matthews, 1985). There is a wealth of literature available examining the aids available to people with poor vision and this will obviously have its uses. It would be tempting in some cases to assume that the visual disturbances will be short-lived and therefore there is no need to go to the effort of getting the adapted equipment. However, MS is unpredictable and visual disturbance is very disruptive to one's life style, therefore action should be taken immediately. Some social work departments have social workers who specialize in helping the blind and partially sighted and will be able to give details of all that is available. The safety aspects of sensory loss are important to assess, e.g. in terms of knowing how hot something is, whether obstacles block a path, or whether a position is giving discomfort. There are other irritating consequences such as dropping things, and being unable to carry out fine manipulative finger movements because sensation is lost in the finger tips.

Another physical disturbance that occurs is the loss of balance. Clearly things such as poor sight and numbness or weakness in the legs can contribute to this. Poor balance can cause problems in many daily activities and can have wide-reaching consequences such as not being able to carry things or go out for fear of falling over. A mother may be unhappy about handling her baby through fear of falling over with it. This is obviously a problem where some degree of help may be required. Whatever help is accepted, for whatever reason, the people involved should discuss all decisions with the patient, e.g. how to organize the house, or look after the children, until some sort of understanding is achieved. This gives the patient a sense of control over the situation. The same principle applies to the nurse. No referral should be made without the agreement of the patient, who should be allowed to state what sort of help is required.

Skin integrity

Poor mobility, numbness, difficulty in feeding, incontinence – these are some of the factors that can threaten the skin integrity of the individual with MS. The result may be soreness, possible infection of cuts and excoriated areas, bruising and pressure sores. Much research-based literature is available to the nurse as to the nature and prevention of pressure sores (David, 1982; Chapman and Chapman, 1986; Gould, 1986). However there is a lack of supported information as to the best ways of treating pressure sores once they occur. The emphasis should therefore be on prevention and the identification of those individuals most at risk of developing pressure sores.

Pressure sores are caused by prolonged pressure, usually over a bony prominence, thereby stopping the blood flow to an area of tissue. It has been estimated that if this pressure is exerted for over two hours then damage to that area of tissue will result. The damage to the tissue is usually deep rooted and so by the time visible signs appear on the skin surface, e.g. redness, broken skin, great damage has already occurred. Therefore the simplest principle in the prevention of pressure sores is that an area of skin should not be sat or lain on for more than two hours at a time, and the individual's position should be changed this frequently. This is a normal activity for healthy people who are never actually sitting or lying completely still. The person who has MS may have lost this protective behaviour for various reasons. Firstly, reduced mobility especially if there is also weakness in both arms, thereby stopping individuals raising themselves by their arms to release pressure. Such a person has to rely on someone else, or on some mechanical means, to relieve pressure. Secondly, there may be numbness to the area of pressure so that the warning feeling of discomfort which signals

Figure 9.3 Factors influencing the risk of pressure sores.

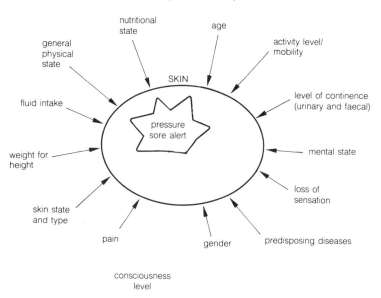

most of us to change position is absent. Thirdly, other sensations such as tingling and pain may mask the feeling of discomfort. Fourthly, the individual may be able to alter position, but the effort is too great to do it as often as is required without assistance.

Several tools, known as pressure sore risk calculators, have been devised to help identify individuals who are most at risk from pressure sores (Waterlow, 1985; Barrett, 1987). They aim to identify a variety of risk factors and measure these to produce a numerical assessment. The actual figure derived from the use of the scale will identify whether or not the individual is at risk. These scales can be easily used in either the community or hospital, and because of their numerical nature, can easily monitor changes in the patient's ability to prevent pressure sores with the fluctuations of the MS. These factors identified by the scales are shown in Figure 9.3. Not all the factors (e.g. gender) are considered in every scale and all the scales need further testing. They are merely a tool to help, and the nurse still has to use her judgement based on knowledge of the individual patient and the factors involved, to make the final decision regarding risk (Barrett, 1987).

In hospital, staff should be available to help move patients at regular intervals. In the community, if the individual needs help in changing position, there needs to be a support network available to help the individual move. It is unlikely that community nurses can call every two hours. Relatives or friends, if involved, need to be taught safe lifting techniques, and thought needs to be given to appropriate equipment either to help the individual move, e.g. hoists, or to help relieve pressure from vulnerable sites. Boore *et al.* (1987; p.563) list many of the pressure relieving products currently available. Again the occupational therapist and the physiotherapist, together with the aids department, will be able to help. ARMS, the MS Society, the Tissue Viability Society, the Disabled Living Foundation and other specialist groups are also good sources of equipment and advice.

Restricted mobility can bring with it other problems as well as pressure sores. Frustration and depression are common reactions, and if the individual is unable to get out and about, social isolation can develop. There are also physical risks of thrombosis, urinary tract infections, renal stasis, joint contractures and chest infections (see Chapter 4).

Fatigue

This physical disturbance very much affects all aspects of life. Extreme tiredness is a common symptom of MS and is usually unpredictable in nature. Difficulties with mobility and movement may exacerbate it. It is easy for relatives and the professionals to underestimate the level of fatigue, and its disruptive effect on activity. The fatigue is such that even a small activity, like pegging out the washing, requires a rest period after. Rest will usually ease the sense of fatigue and adequate rest periods should be scheduled to meet energy demands. If energy must be expended to a great degree on one day, then rest must be made available both before and after. Plans are difficult to make in advance but energy can be budgeted to try and ensure that the fatigue level is low when necessary. As many team members, both in hospital and in the community, will want to plan activities with the patient, liaison and planning between all concerned are important. The nurse is probably best placed to act as coordinator in consultation with the patient.

If the patient is unaware of the reason for this fatigue, it will be difficult to organize life accordingly. Similarly, because the symptom is not visible, close friends, partners, children, etc., may be intolerant of the disruption it can cause to plans, or of the fact that the individual is always tired. They need adequate information to develop appropriate understanding so that their life can also be structured.

Psychological and social implications

The emphasis on nursing models looking at the whole person means that psychological and social implications of MS must also be considered. Any chronic illness leads to a change in activity levels and often requires a readjustment in personal goals. However well adapted the individual may have become to living with MS, there will still be times when he becomes frustrated at not being able to do something or go somewhere, at having to rely on others for help, and at not being able to move about or see clearly. This is where the need for that independent listener is so important.

It is accepted that individuals have a variety of physical problems depending on which nerve pathways are currently affected. These in turn will cause possible disruption to social functioning and lead to some emotional and psychological difficulties. It is important to ascertain in the assessment the nature of the individual's mood and to determine the cause of it. Communication of mood, however, may be impaired by speech and visual disturbances. The disabling aspects of the disease can cause frustration and depression. Clearly the mood is caused by the disease to some extent, but not in the way described in most nursing textbooks. Some drug therapies, e.g. steroids, can also cause mood changes. The individual's mood may also be affected by events not connected with MS. In all dealings with individuals with MS it is important to find the cause for what is apparent, and to bear in mind that other events and other diseases can also be the cause of symptoms in the individual, and not just the MS.

Inevitably any change in body functioning and sensations, and their subsequent effects on life style and ability to carry out activities, can result in a change of self-image, perceived self-worth and self-confidence. The nurse can help by emphasizing the importance of putting things into perspective, and providing the individual with sufficient help to achieve personal goals.

The social implications of the disease hinge around the ability to maintain relationships and role functions. Social isolation can occur when the patient feels unable to play his part and therefore feel a burden. It may be just that the effort of getting somewhere alone means that there is little energy left to participate in group activity. Offers of transport may mean that the individual can be a productive member of the group again. The MS patient needs to feel that he has something to contribute, and if others refuse this contribution there may be reluctance to accept other offers of help. In our society we tend to return favours, and people with MS need to feel that they can do the same to keep relationships properly balanced. The social circle of any individual with MS includes many groups, and the individual may require help from the community nurse to explain to some of these groups the nature of MS.

The fluctuating nature of the disease may make holding down a job difficult but, as has been seen, many do continue to work. The occupational health nurse can play a part in increasing understanding from employers and colleagues. In some cases the work may be easier to achieve than the alternative, e.g. a young mother may find that she can budget her energy better and carry out a 'normal role' by working and employing someone else to perform the bulk of child-care. Within the house, adaptations may be made and labour-saving devices introduced. However, the biggest barrier to most of these may be financial. As with any disabling condition the levels of benefits available are dwindling, but those available can be used beneficially, e.g. mobility allowance enables the purchase of an adapted car and this can reduce social isolation and save energy.

Dying

The final aspect of any life style will always be the way that we die. MS is not generally expected to be a cause of death, and most people with MS actually die from factors associated with MS rather than the MS itself (Matthews *et al.*, 1985). The extra strain put on the body system from all the effects of the disease may well increase the individual's susceptibility to these fatal causes, hence the importance of developing a health promoting and illness preventing approach to care. There is an ever increasing wealth of material concerned with the dying, the place of death (hospital or home), and the roles of those involved. The positive message of health promotion concerning the areas of health most at risk of developing fatal problems should be emphasized, thereby giving individuals the means by which to try and control their situation. Other disease processes cannot be excluded and so a general positive approach to health is advisable.

When the person with MS is dying, the nurse will need to be involved with both the individual and the family. Sims (1988) discusses how people cope with dying and the various stages they go through. She emphasizes the need for patients to be involved in their own care, where possible, supported by the family. Elder (1976) describes how each family will have its own beliefs and views regarding death, and Assel (1976) discusses the strategies that can be used by the nurse to assist the patient and family at this time. The nurse should continue to support the family after the patient has died. To be able to do this, the nurse must also be supported. The community nurse in particular may be isolated, and colleague support networks need to be established. The practical care of the dying person will depend on the cause of death, but will involve providing physical comfort and dignity, and a continuation of life's normal activities as far as possible.

Nurses have a breadth of knowledge and a wide range of skills that can be offered to the individual who has MS as part of health promoting care. MS presents many problems to both patient and nurse, but as this chapter has demonstrated, by working in a partnership, many of these can be tackled in such a way as to assist the patient to lead the life of his choice.

REFERENCES

Assel, R.A. (1976) If you were dying, in *Dealing with Death and Dying*, Nursing Skill Book. Intermed Communications, Jenkintown, Pa.

Barrett, E. (1987) Putting risk calculators in their place. *Nursing Times,* Feb. 18, 65–70.

Boore, J.R.P., Champion, R. and Ferguson, M.C. (1987) *Nursing the Physically Ill Adult.* Churchill Livingstone, Edinburgh.

Boore, J. (1980) Normal and abnormal micturition. *Nursing. The add-on journal of clinical nursing,* October, 763–5.

Burnfield, A. (1985) *Multiple Sclerosis: A personal exploration.* Souvenir Press, (E and A) Ltd., London.

Catanzaro, M. (1980) Nursing care of the person with multiple sclerosis. *American Journal of Nursing,* **80**, 286–91.

Chapman, E.J. and Chapman, R. (1986) Treatment of pressure sores: the state of the art, in *Clinical Nursing Practice* (ed. A.J. Tierney). Churchill Livingstone, London.

CURN Project (1982) *Clean Intermittent Catheterization.* Grune and Stratton, New York.

David, J.A. (1982) Pressure sore treatment: a literature review. *International Journal of Nursing Studies,* **19**(4), 183–91.

Davis, M.Z. (1984) Nursing and the chronically ill patient in the acute-care setting. *Journal of Advanced Nursing,* **9**, 257–66.

Elder, R.G. (1976) Dying and society, in *Dealing with Death and Dying,* Nursing Skill Book. Intermed Communications, Jenkintown, Pa.

Ewles, L. and Simnett, I. (1985) *Promoting Health.* John Wiley and Sons, Chichester.

Forsythe, E. (1988) *Multiple Sclerosis. Exploring Sickness and Health.* Faber and Faber, London.

Glew, J. (1986) A woman's lot? *Nursing Times,* April 9, 69–71.

Glower, D., Thomas, T., North, W. *et al.* (1986) Urinary symptoms and sexual difficulties. *Nursing Times,* 9 April, 72–5.

Gorman, E., Rudd, A. and Ebers, G.C. (1984) Giving the diagnosis of multiple sclerosis, in *The Diagnosis of Multiple Sclerosis* (eds C.M. Poser *et al.*). Thieme-Stratton, Inc., New York.

Gould, D. (1986) Pressure sore prevention and treatment: an example of nurses' failure to implement research. *Journal of Advanced Nursing,* **11**, 389–94.

Graham, J. (1987) *Multiple Sclerosis. A Self-help Guide to its Management.* Thorsons Publishing Group, Wellingborough.

Hanson, S.M.H. (1987) Family nursing and chronic illness, in *Families and Chronic Illness* (eds L.M. Wright and M. Leahey). Springhouse Corporation, Springhouse, Pennslyvania.

Kratz, C.R. (1980) *Care of the Longterm Sick in the Community.* Churchill Livingstone, Edinburgh.

Lechtenberg, R. (1988) *Multiple Sclerosis Fact Book.* F.A. Davis Company, Philadelphia.

Levin, L.S. (1978) Patient education and self-care: how do they differ? *Nursing Outlook,* March, 170–5.

Long, B.C. and Phipps, W.J. (1985) *Essentials of Medical–Surgical Nursing. A nursing process approach.* C.V. Mosby Co., St Louis.

Maanen, H.M.Th. van (1981) Rehabilitation: core of nursing. *International Nursing Review,* **28**(1), 9–14.

McClymont, M.E. (1985) Intervention and care in long term nursing of the adult, in *Long Term Care* (ed. K. King). Churchill Livingstone, Edinburgh.

McDonnell, M., Hentgen, J., Holland, N. *et al.* (1980) MS: Problem orientated nursing care plans. *American Journal of Nursing,* Feb., 292–7.

Matthews, W.B. (1985) Symptoms and signs, in *McAlpine's Multiple Sclerosis* (eds W.B. Matthews, E.D. Acheson, J.R. Batchelor *et al.*). Churchill Livingstone, London, pp. 96–145.

Matthews, W.B., Acheson, E.D., Batchelor, J.R. *et al.* (1985) *McAlpine's Multiple Sclerosis.* Churchill Livingstone, Edinburgh.

Norton, C. (1986) Nursing the incontinent patient, in *Clinical Nursing Practice* (A.J. Tierney). Churchill Livingstone, Edinburgh.

Orem, D.E. (1980) *Nursing: Concepts of Practice.* McGraw-Hill, New York.

Price, G. (1980) MS. The challenge to the family. *American Journal of Nursing,* Feb., 282–5.

Roper, N., Logan, W. and Tierney, A. (1980) *The Elements of Nursing.* Churchill Livingstone, Edinburgh.

Roy, C. (1976) *Introduction to Nursing: An adaptation model.* Prentice Hall, New Jersey.

Sims, S. (1988) Coping with dying, in *Nursing Issues and Research in Terminal Care* (eds J. Wilson-Barnett and J. Raiman). John Wiley and Sons, Chichester.

Slater, R.J. and Yearwood, A.C. (1980) MS: Facts, faith and hope. *American Journal of Nursing,* Feb., 276-81.

Smith, N.K.G. (1988) Continence Advisory Services in England. *Health Trends,* **20**, 22-3.

Smithers, K. (1988) Practical problems of mothers who have multiple sclerosis. *Midwife, Health Visitor and Community Nurse,* **24**(5), 165-8.

Stockwell, F. (1984) *The Unpopular Patient.* Croom Helm, London.

Thomas, T.M., Karran, O.D. and Meade, T.W. (1981) Management of urinary incontinence in patients with multiple sclerosis. *Journal of the Royal College of General Practitioners,* **31**(226), 296-8.

Ulrich, S.P., Canale, S.W. and Wendell, S.A. (1986) *Nursing Care Planning Guides. A nursing diagnosis approach.* W.B. Saunders Co., Philadelphia.

Waterlow, J. (1985) A risk assessment card. *Nursing Times,* November 27, 49-52.

Webb, C. (1985) *Sexuality, Nursing and Health.* John Wiley and Sons, Chichester.

Wilson, J. and Roe, B. (1986) Nursing management of patients with an indwelling urethral catheter, in *Clinical Nursing Practice* (ed. A.J. Tierney). Churchill Livingstone, Edinburgh.

Wilson-Barnett, J. (ed.) (1983) *Patient Teaching.* Churchill Livingstone, Edinburgh.

10

Personal and social meanings of multiple sclerosis

Judith Monks

Health professionals, together with people who have multiple sclerosis, recognize MS as a medical condition with associated pathological features giving rise to particular signs and symptoms. This is the most widely held view of what the term 'multiple sclerosis' means. Yet the value we place on biomedicine often leads us to suppose that medical descriptions are the only valid descriptions, with respect to the current state of knowledge. In one sense this must be so, for MS is essentially a medical term. Unlike a 'chill', for example, the condition must be formally diagnosed before legitimate claim may be made to it. What is less obvious is that medical descriptions of MS are just that, i.e. descriptions, and like any others, identify particular sets of problems for particular purposes. The increasingly narrow focus of medical research on specific organs or systems, and the continuing endeavour to demonstrate physical disorder visually (by scanning, for example) and through precise measurement, are particular ways of making MS 'concrete' and therefore manageable. Where the detailed physiological disorder is understood, it is reasoned, specific treatments may be effectively targeted.

If, for the moment, we regard the medical description of MS as just one type of description with its own purposes and its own ways of defining the problems requiring management, we may also appreciate other formulations, equally valid though differently focused. Gubrium's (1986) work on Alzheimer's disease is relevant here. He analysed descriptions of the condition provided by nurses, and other caregivers, and showed how these reflected the problems of each group in providing care. He also showed how the descriptions were structured according to concern with 'amelioration' or 'tribulation' and how the precarious distinction between Alzheimer's disease and ageing required repeated reinforcement (Gubrium, 1986; pp. 3–9, 16–20). Gubrium's reasoning applied equally to descriptions of MS where medical facts and problems may take second place to other concerns. The quality and variability of the meaning of MS to those with the condition themselves may be appreciated from the growing number of personal accounts (Birrer 1979; Brown, 1984; Lowry, 1984; Davoud, 1985) and from research which has sought to present the experience of MS from a personal viewpoint (Cunningham, 1977; Wynne, 1982; Robinson, 1988a). Robinson (1988a) particularly points to problems in sustaining an understanding of MS as a discrete condition in the face of vague, ambiguous symptoms.

This chapter considers work which has shed light on the range of meanings which MS may hold for those who are personally affected. It looks first at what is involved in interpreting initial symptoms and establishing the diagnosis as a personally significant label around which meanings may be constructed. Secondly, it discusses some apparently common meanings of the 'MS' label itself, and aspects of the disease's particular manifestations. Thirdly, day-to-day life with MS is considered with respect to personal relationships, income and employment. It is not the intention here to provide a catalogue of experiences and understandings which represent the typical meaning of MS for those affected, for meanings will in many ways be individual. The aim is rather to indicate some of the ways in which those individual meanings may be shaped. Lastly, some of the implications of such meanings for patients' expectations of therapy, and their influences on the relationship between therapist and patient, will be discussed.

ACHIEVING THE DIAGNOSIS: ESTABLISHING THE MEANING OF PHYSICAL DISORDER

In Stewart and Sullivan's (1982) study of 60 people with MS, the diagnosis 'was seldom easily or rapidly reached', taking an 'average of five and half years for the individuals to be correctly diagnosed' (1982; p.1399). This often lengthy and problematic prediagnostic period is critical for it is during this time that 'multiple sclerosis' becomes significant for the person affected. The way in which such significance develops carries implications for how the diagnosis is received and accepted, and subsequently how living with MS is approached.

It is worth emphasizing that the initial symptoms of MS may be transient and undramatic, and indeed not recognized as symptoms at all but simply as normal health deviations, easily explained in terms of a person's situation. It is not until symptoms have become pronounced, for instance by their duration, visibility or interference with activities in daily life, that a doctor will usually be consulted. This event may follow many weeks or months of uncertainty about health status, involving discussions with family, friends and work colleagues about whether anything is 'really' wrong (Cunningham, 1977; pp. 22–3; Robinson, 1988a; pp. 14–19). Thus by the time of their initial medical consultation, many people are already likely to hold ideas about the meaning of their symptoms and will be looking for confirmation of these ideas, or for arbitration where they conflict with the views of others. Where totally perplexed, they will be seeking a full explanation.

The nature of MS symptoms often makes expectations, such as those described above, hard to meet. The available medical 'slots' within the doctor's frame of reference may not easily accommodate the vague and rather unusual sensations and experiences which patients often attempt to express (Monks, 1986; pp. 3–5). In the very early stages, both patient and doctor may agree that 'nothing is wrong' but later when, in the patient's view, complaints continue to be dismissed, frustration may lead to a series of consultations with different specialists and often also to a personal search for information and a process of self-diagnosis. During this phase symptoms may be misinterpreted and incorrect conclusions made or feared (Stewart and Sullivan, 1982; p.1400).

There is evidence that the quest for diagnosis is often a period of considerable trauma. It may be accompanied by uncertainty about the potential seriousness of what may be wrong, and frequently also by doubts about whether anything is wrong at all. These uncertainties carry implications for faith in one's own mental status and for relationships with others. Thus an eventual diagnosis of MS, while unwelcome, often ill-understood and sometimes unexpected, may also be received with some relief. At the point of diagnosis then, 'MS' is as significant for what it is *not* (e.g. a life-threatening condition), as much as for what it is, and most importantly for its being *something*. The increase in both social and medical support after diagnosis and the practical usefulness and psychological comfort of a legitimate explanation of symptoms have been frequently noted (Cunningham, 1977; p.30; Stewart and Sullivan, 1982; p.1402); Robinson, 1988a; p.30).

Unfortunately, in spite of the positive value of a diagnostic label now being more widely recognized, it seems that many doctors continue to delay telling patients of their suspicions, and in some cases may inform only a close relative or indeed never offer a diagnosis at all. Recent studies by Robinson (1983; p.9) and Elian and Dean (1985; p.27) have suggested that up to one third of patients will have guessed or discovered the diagnosis for themselves before they are formally told. Therapists and other health professionals may sometimes be implicated in the gradual process of enlightenment, or unwittingly instrumental in actual disclosure.

Whatever the circumstances in which the diagnosis is learned, in the first instance it is likely to be the medical aspects which are stressed in any explanations. Doctors may tell as much as they can about the nature of the physical disorder and the possibility of treatment, but uncertainty of medical prognosis will make discussions of functional limitation and wider implications more difficult. Therefore, at diagnosis, while a person may for the first time be able to make sense of their physical disorder, they may have little opportunity to discuss the wider aspects of their situation. Often they will ask themselves 'Why me?' and 'Why now?', and seek to explain the occurrence of their illness in terms of their general philosophy of life. They will often also try to assess the implications of the diagnosis, of now being a 'person with MS', for their personal past, present and future. These are problems which medical science can address only partially, for someone's body is not only a physical unit, but also has a personal presence in the world in which they live, and forms an integral part of their selfhood. Physical disorder, particularly when it is established in a medical diagnosis, thus demands a reinterpretation of a person's self-concept and relationship with the world around them. It is this new sense of self and of being in the world which carry the personal and social meanings of MS.

THE SIGNIFICANCE AND CONSEQUENCES OF LIVING WITH MS

The meaning of MS to the person concerned may be considered in terms of their changed relationship, both with themselves, through their new self-concept, and with the outside world. These separate domains of meaning broadly relate to Bury's (1988) notions of 'meaning as significance' and 'meaning as consequence', and it is under these headings that the personal and social meanings of MS will be discussed.

143

Meaning as significance

Bury (1988) points out that being ill, and particularly being recognized by others as ill, can have a significance quite apart from what might be considered as the consequence, although the particular significance of an illness may carry consequences of its own. Illnesses vary in the type and import of their significance. For example, the common cold may signify little other than the mild irresponsibility of the person who catches it, while other conditions, such as cancer or AIDS, are highly charged emotionally. MS has a number of features which appear particularly significant for those affected.

The potential severity of MS together with other implications, discussed below, usually seems to require a holistic explanation for its occurrence. The person who has MS needs to make sense of the fact in terms of who they believe themselves to be and how they have arrived at their identity. This often involves a life review focusing on events and situations to which the person sees themselves to have related in a specific way. For example, there may have been contact with substances possibly significant in the onset of MS, as suggested by the clinical ecology approach to aetiology (Birrer, 1979). Alternatively, past situations might have been psychologically stressful, or perhaps there were aspects of the person's social position or of their relationship with their deity which might have been relevant. By considering such possibilities the person is able to build up a picture of their situation which is rational to themselves, and they may also be able to work through feelings of responsibility for their MS and begin to plan for self-management (Wynne, 1982; pp. 5–7; Robinson, 1988a; pp. 78–80). Williams (1984) has called these explanatory life reviews 'narrative reconstructions' and has drawn attention to their focus on the impact of the illness and changes in personal and social circumstances, rather than the disease process itself. Life reviews thus not only explain but confer meaning on illness.

Biographical reviews and associated explanations of illness are modified over time to take account of new developments in the course of the illness and of knowledge gained from other sources. Thus explanations are not stable, and neither are they necessarily held one at a time. A person may recognize a number of different explanations for their MS, each consistent within its own frame of reference, in much the same way that a medical scientist might recognize both genetic and environmental 'causes'. Since different concerns are reflected in these various understandings they may on the surface appear contradictory. In Birrer's (1979) account, for example, one can note the interchange between reflection on MS as 'a functional disorder of ecological relationships', an explanation which focuses on an environmental aetiology, and the metaphysical description of MS as 'a peculiar and characteristic mode of being in the world'. The range of personal and medical explanations which may be employed by someone with MS are thus complementary, serving different purposes and answering different questions.

Apart from it biographical significance, MS often carries a number of other meanings which relate to its general nature as a chronic and potentially severely disabling condition, and to its specific manifestations. Again these meanings should not be seen as static, carrying a one-to-one relationship with the relevant MS characteristic, but as emerging and developing over the course of the illness. On a general level MS frequently seems to be associated with a sense of loss and therefore perhaps resolvable through a process of grieving stages or phases of adjustment have been described, each with its characteristic 'response' such as denial, anger, and acceptance. Not all people with MS are expected to pass through every stage, nor in sequence, although the style of adaptation during any one period is invariably represented as stable (Matson and Brooks, 1977; pp.249–50; Gorman, Rudd and Ebers, 1984; p.218; VanderPlate, 1984; pp.263–7). The notion of adjustment stages has been popular in clinical practice for it has provided a framework which practitioners may use to monitor their patient's progress. Other work, however, has suggested that this model might be inappropriate as it allows for little individual variation and minimizes the importance of a person's social circumstances (Oliver, 1983).

Specific features of MS also convey particular meanings, especially those associated with physical disability and a need for aids or personal help.

These meanings are generally considered to be negative, being associated with self-devaluation and stagmatization. Duval (1984) refers to a complex of negative feelings associated with MS symptoms which she calls 'distress' and suggests that these are constituted and expressed in ways which reflect general cultural values. Thus, in American society at least, the loss of independence, mobility and predictability of life may become the most significant features of the illness. Others frequently cite incontinence and the use of a wheelchair as symbolizing regression to an infantile state coupled with extreme dependency (Cunningham, 1977; Wynne, 1982; Robinson, 1988a).

145

Meaning as consequence

Those involved in the care of people with MS often find it useful to think separately about the disease and its consequences, for this allows for the possibility of intervention in order to modify the consequences, where treatment of the disease process itself is not available.

The consequences of MS which have received most attention concern psychological reactions (discussed above), interpersonal relationships, employment and income. A full review of each of these areas is not possible here, the aim being rather to provide an overview indicating the range of consequences of MS which are currently recognized.

Concern for interpersonal relationships stems from the recognition of the crucial role of social interaction for the maintenance of self-concept. Interest has been directed therefore towards the effect of MS both on the quality of social relationships, and on their availability which may be diminished through disability or fear of rejection. Certain manifestations of MS, such as particular symptoms or the use of aids, may carry negative values, and interactions with others may therefore have to be 'managed' to minimize their potentially damaging effects, or even in order for interaction to take place at all. One management strategy might be to limit social relationships as far as possible to those with others in a similar situation, for example by forming new friendships through a self-help group. Other strategies include attempts to hide symptoms from visibility or defuse their emotional impact by treating them as routine (Strauss, 1975; Cunningham, 1977; Miles, 1979).

Further to this concern for the quality of social relationships is one for their requisite psychosocial and material resources. Personality, the availability of social support and an adequate income, for example, have all been seen as part of the context in which life with MS develops. The source of social support most commonly studied has been that provided by the family. 'Family' is a concept the meaning of which has been generally taken for granted by those who have used it, but implicitly it has referred to a lived-in or otherwise 'close' social unit, members of which, through their interlocking roles and intensity of interaction, have been seen to provide mutually for the establishment of self-identity.

Thus the consequences of MS are not confined to the person directly affected, and indeed families themselves have been said to 'have MS' with associated needs for grieving, explanation and information (Gorman *et al.*, 1984; Burnfield, 1985). The implications for family members are discussed in detail in Chapter 11. In view of the acknowledged crucial role of the family in shaping the personal consequences of MS, and also of the apparently high divorce and separation rate (Robinson, 1988b), it is perhaps surprising that such little attention has been paid to the social relationships of those without close relatives. At most, there has been discussion of 'friendship' in general and here concern has been with problematic and diminishing relationships. The role of close friends and the consequences of MS for the quality of friendships, particularly where these are more significant for the person involved than family relationships, remain largely unresearched.

The other major area in which the consequences of MS have been studied is that of employment. Opportunities for appropriate paid employment have been seen as important in that they provide for social intercourse and serve as a basis for the establishment of self-identity. More materialistically they are also seen as a source of finance to enhance the general quality of life and meet the extra demands of illness and disability. Research in this field has indicated that people with MS are more likely than the general population to be underemployed or unemployed, but also that this cannot be regarded as a direct reflection of physical disablement or the psychological status of the person affected. Just as important are discriminatory practices and lack of flexibility within the employment sector, constraints related to the other social roles of the person involved, and environmental problems, such as those related to transport and access to buildings (Elian and Dean, 1985; Kornblith, LaRocca and Baum, 1986; Robinson, 1988a).

Lack of suitable employment thus seems a commonly experienced consequence of MS although, unfortunately, the processes involved are still barely understood. Similarly, although people disabled by MS, like other disabled people, seem to have a lower average income than the general population, the ways in which this may come about have received little attention (Locker, 1983). A contributing factor appears to be that many of those eligible do not claim their full complement of financial allowances. Elian and Dean (1985) have shown that this may be due to people's lack of awareness of the existence of such allowances, or of their entitlements, or even their diagnosis. Genevie, Kallos and Struening (1987) have drawn attention to the way in which a variety of needs are reduced by an adequate income, thus underlining its general significance.

147

PERSONAL AND SOCIAL MEANINGS: IMPLICATIONS FOR THERAPY

How, from such diverse implications, does one extract what MS 'really means'? This is an important question because the meaning of MS in terms of explanation, significance and consequences carries implications for the types of therapy which will be sought, or understood and accepted. The vast literature on non-compliance with medical advice has indicated how the understandings and goals of health professional and patient might not always coincide (Conrad, 1985).

Much of the writing on compliance has focused on the personal characteristics of patients, especially their health-related beliefs and understanding of medical instructions, and the affective relationship between patient and doctor, or therapist. Satisfaction of patients with medical consultations has claimed particular attention because of its consistent association with acceptance of medical advice. Studies of patient satisfaction (Cartwright, 1983; pp.99–113) are, however, increasingly criticized for assuming that health problems may be defined and dealt with solely in terms of medical knowledge. Patients' ideas, it is said, are explored only with a view to modification or correction. The alternative view proposed by some authors accepts patients' understandings as valid within their own frame of reference, and focuses on the articulation of these understandings with health professionals, noting how patients' satisfaction may be produced through the coincidence of similar ideas, or negotiation on an equal basis (Fitzpatrick and Hopkins, 1981; Tuckett et al., 1985). In addition, some studies have investigated how people do manage their illnesses by integrating personal and prescribed regimens, thus presenting non-compliance in a more positive light. Conrad (1985), for example, in his research on living with epilepsy, concluded that self-regulation of medication (which in some cases involved stopping drugs altogether for a period) established a sense of control over what otherwise seemed to be an unpredictable and ill-understood condition. Respondents both increased their drug dosage to deal with practical circumstances, and reduced it to test the effects. Many disliked their dependence on drugs and the confirmation of their epileptic state which medication provided, and therefore sought to reduce dosage to a minimum. Some people with diabetes have been found to take a similar approach to their diet and insulin therapy (Kelleher, 1988).

One of the achievements of this more recent work on compliance and management is to indicate how meanings of illness are drawn from its relationship with everyday life. Literature recognizably 'about' MS has by definition brought MS into focus. Through this literature MS is seen as an entity to be managed, and particular targeted regimens as essential to this management. However, as indicated by the work of Conrad (1985) and Kelleher (1988) and also by autobiographical accounts such as those mentioned earlier, disease does not necessarily retain this status away from the clinic. It may become conceptually less discrete, representing no more than one aspect of a life in which priorities remain similar to those prevailing before diagnosis but to which bodily disorder now adds a particular quality.

Recognition that MS and its management might not receive a high profile in daily life may seem to pose problems for those who teach patients management skills or prescribe regimens. However, to be aware of how MS slips in and out of the focus of someone's attention according to circumstances, is to be aware of the differences between formally prescribed regimens and methods of management which harmonize with everyday living. Transformation of one into the other is not simply a question of practicalities. Therapy as such, or the dependency implicit in direct nursing care, may be an unwelcome intrusion *per se*, reinforcing the sick status as well as hindering activities. For example, a diet conceived in formal terms, may be a constant reminder of illness both to the person taking it and to observers. A redefinition of the diet as 'healthy eating' may carry no such implications, although it might be associated with a kind of 'healthism' which may or may not be acceptable. Conversely, and still in relation to diet, a disliked food such as liver may be eaten far more readily as 'medicine' than as 'food', but the person involved must be able and willing to make such a shift in perspective and the rationale for doing so must be meaningful. The desirable therapeutic goal, therefore, may be one of satisfactory living within the context of MS rather than managing MS as such. This is a view which invites exploration of the circumstances in which symptoms or other problems either become or cease to be apparent, and in which formal strategies either may or may not be felt appropriate. Using the flexible approach which this implies, health professional and patient together may examine the various ways in which specific aspects of MS might be accommodated.

'Multiple sclerosis' may, therefore, carry a range of meanings. These include not only meanings derived from a biomedical perspective but also those related to the significance of MS for a person's self-concept and view of their relationship with the world. Other meanings relate to the consequences of having MS in terms of roles, activities and social relationships. Such meanings carry implications for therapy and care which relate both to the definition of those problems requiring attention, and to appropriate ways of tackling them. Much of the literature available in this area has been criticized for its tendency to identify difficulties which require targeted management, and hence its inability to interpret apparently satisfactory modes of living as anything other than examples of 'adjustment' or 'coping'. An alternative view is that a life style associated with disability or chronic illness is normal, if somewhat unusual, and needs placing in appropriate prospective (Shearer, 1981; Oliver, 1983).

Of course people with MS talk readily of problems and management strategies when invited to do so, although they also, as noted above, sometimes provide very different accounts. It was argued earlier that people's perspectives on MS may change according to the aspect of life at the focus of their attention. In some circumstances the use of formal strategies to manage MS, or one of its associated problems, may seem quite appropriate while in others different concerns are paramount. It was suggested that therapists, nurses and people with MS might work together in planning how best to accommodate the illness. A basis for such mutual understanding and cooperation between health professionals and people with MS can indeed be found in the methods both use to define goals and seek to achieve them. As has been explained, people with MS deal with symptoms in both formal and less directed *ad hoc* ways. Health workers also draw on more than theoretical knowledge in solving their own professional problems. In fact, in most interactions between therapists and patients theory may provide only a general background against which practical decisions are made, past patients providing a resource of knowledge for those treated subsequently (Gubrium and Buckholt, 1982; p.45). This is why professional experience is so valuable. Although theory can be brought to bear on difficult problems, much work is accomplished, with the aid of experience, by attention to more immediate concerns, in other words, particular achievements with particular patients. This reflection on professional work can provide insight into the 'work' involved in living with chronic illness. Here 'theoretical' concerns with disease, symptoms and therapy also forms only one orientation, which may be employed far less frequently away from the clinical setting. The meaning of multiple sclerosis evident when health professional and patient interact, while particular and focused, does therefore provide a starting point for uncovering other meanings and for tailoring management appropriately.

REFERENCES

Birrer, C. (1979) *Multiple Sclerosis: A personal view.* Charles C. Thomas, Springfield, Illinois.

Brown, J. (1984) One man's experience with multiple sclerosis, in *Multiple Sclerosis: Psychological and Social Aspects.* (ed. A.F. Simons). Heinemann, London, 21–9.

Burnfield, A. (1985) *Multiple Sclerosis: A personal exploration.* Souvenir Press, London.

Bury, M. (1988) Meanings at risk: the experience of arthritis, in *Living with Chronic Illness.* (eds R. Anderson and M. Bury). Unwin Hyman, London.

Cartwright, A. (1983) *Health Surveys in Practice and Potential: A Critical Review of their Scope and Methods.* King Edward's Hospital Fund for London, London.

Conrad, P. (1985) The meaning of medications: another look at compliance. *Social Science and Medicine,* **20**(1), 29–37.

Cunningham, D.J. (1977) Stigma and social isolation: self-perceived problems of a group of multiple sclerosis sufferers. HSRU Report 27, Health Services Research Unit, University of Kent.

Davoud, N. (1985) *Where Do I Go From Here?* Piatkus Books, London.

Duval, M.L. (1984) Psychosocial metaphors of physical distress among MS patients. *Social Science and Medicine,* **19**(6), 635–8.

Elian, M. and Dean, G. (1985) To tell or not to tell the diagnosis of multiple sclerosis. *Lancet,* **ii**, 27–8.

Fitzpatrick, R.M. and Hopkins, A. (1981) Patients' satisfaction with communication in neurological outpatient clinics. *Journal of Psychosomatic Research,* **25**(5), 329–34.

Genevie, L., Kallos, J.E. and Struening, E.L. (1987) An overview of patients' perceptions of their needs: multiple sclerosis as a paradigm. *Journal of Neurologic Rehabilitation,* **1**(1), 9–12.

Gorman, E., Rudd, A. and Ebers, G.C. (1984) Giving the diagnosis of multiple sclerosis, in *The Diagnosis of Multiple Sclerosis* (eds E.M. Poser, D.W. Paty, L.C. Scheinberg *et al.*). Thieme-Stratton, New York, 216–22.

Gubrium, J.F. and Buckholdt, D.R. (1982) Describing care: image and practice in rehabilitation. Oelgeschlager, Gunn and Hain Publishers Inc., Cambridge, Mass.

Gubrium, J.F. (1986) *Oldtimers and Alzheimers: The descriptive organization of senility.* JAI Press, Greenwich, Connecticut.

Kelleher, D. (1988) Coming to terms with diabetes: coping strategies and non-compliance, in *Living with Chronic Illness.* (eds R. Anderson and M. Bury). Unwin Hyman, London.

Kornblith, A.B., LaRocca, N.G. and Baum, H.M. (1986) Employment in individuals with multiple sclerosis. *International Journal of Rehabilitation Research,* **9**(2), 155–65.

Locker, D. (1983) *Disability and Disadvantage. The Consequences of Chronic Illness.* Tavistock Publications, New York.

Lowry, F. (1984) One woman's experience with multiple sclerosis, in *Multiple Sclerosis: Psychological and Social Aspects* (ed. A.F. Simons). Heinemann, London, 30–5.

Matson, R.R. and Brooks, N.A. (1977) Adjusting to multiple sclerosis: an exploratory study. *Social Science and Medicine,* **11**, 245–50.

Miles, A. (1979) Some psycho-social consequences of multiple sclerosis: problems of social interaction and group identity. *British Journal of Medical Psychology,* **52**, 321–31.

Monks, J. (1986) Doing justice to MS symptoms. Gen.Report No.5, Brunel-ARMS Research Unit, Brunel, University of West London.

Oliver, M.J. (1983) *Social Work with Disabled People.* Macmillan, London.

Robinson, I. (1983) Discovering the diagnosis of MS. Gen.Report No.3, Brunel-ARMS Research Unit, Brunel, University of West London.

Robinson, I. (1988a) *Multiple Sclerosis.* Routledge, London.

Robinson, I. (1988b) Reconstructing lives: negotiating the meaning of multiple sclerosis, in *Living with Chronic Illness.* (eds R. Anderson and M. Bury). Unwin Hyman, London.

Shearer, A. (1981) *Disability: whose handicap?* Basil Blackwell, Oxford.

Stewart, D.C. and Sullivan, I.J. (1982) Illness behaviour and the sick role in chronic disease: the case of multiple sclerosis. *Social Science and Medicine,* **16**, 1397–404.

Strauss, A.L. (1975) *Chronic Illness and the Quality of Life.* C.V. Mosby Co., St. Louis, USA.

Tuckett, D., Boulton, M., Olson, C. and Williams, A. (1985) *Meetings Between Experts: An approach to sharing ideas in medical consultations.* Tavistock, London.

VanderPlate, C. (1984) Psychological aspects of multiple sclerosis and its treatment: towards a biopsychosocial perspective. *Health Psychology,* **3**(3), 253–72.

Williams, B. (1984) The genesis of chronic illness: narrative reconstruction. *Sociology of Health and Illness,* **6**(2), 175–200.

Wynne, A. (1982) Talking about MS. Gen.Report No.1, Brunel-ARMS Research Unit, Brunel, University of West London.

11

Patients, their families
and multiple sclerosis

Ian Robinson, Rosemary Jones, and Julia Segal

Formal systems of health care, whether in a hospital or a community setting, are largely focused on individuals. Given the emphasis on the physical pathology associated with conditions like multiple sclerosis the primary concern is to seek to remedy individual impairments or functional problems. Unsurprisingly, most professional attention is directed to achieving these remedies through the medium of a one-to-one relationship between the doctor or therapist and the patient. Yet many problems associated with MS have, in addition, a social and a family dimension (see Chapters 1 and 10). This social dimension is significant in a variety of ways for the professional management of the condition.

First, the disease often occurs at a time when critical life decisions are being taken in relation to marriage, furthering careers or having children. Therefore for therapists or other professional advisors understanding and managing the physical effects of the disease will be intricately bound up with the concerns of patients and their families about their personal futures. They will wish to know, or to predict, or at the very least try to understand the consequences of their physical condition for those futures.

Second, most management of MS, as most health care in general, will occur in informal and familial situations, where day-to-day management will be undertaken by family members. Professional advice will be as frequently filtered through the values, attitudes and skills of those family members, as it will be through the patients themselves. Therefore the effectiveness and success of therapies will be partly contingent on appreciating the central role of the family in the management of the condition.

The word 'family' is used in this chapter in a generic way to refer to many different kinds of relationship which may be found in households where there is someone with MS. Sometimes it refers to a wide group of people who are related by marriage or descent to each other, and at other times it refers to members of a household who are living with each other but who may not be formally related in these ways. It is important to recognize that there may be partners of the same as well as the opposite sex. In most of the family situations found in relation to MS concerns, anxieties and difficulties, although expressed in different ways, are fundamentally related to ways of managing the intrusion of this uncertain and problematic condition.

Burnfield expresses the point well about the significance of the family involvement in MS when he says that 'When someone has MS the the whole family has MS as well' (1985; p.95). This should not be taken in a literal sense, but in the sense that all the members of a family are likely to have to come to terms with MS in their relationship with each other, as well as in their feelings about themselves. However, issues may be raised initially about the physical characteristics and consequences of the disease itself and what it might imply for both individual members of a family and the family as a whole.

FAMILIES, THE FUTURE AND THE NATURE OF MULTIPLE SCLEROSIS

When someone discovers that they have MS, or even suspects that this is a possible diagnosis, many questions arise both about their own future and that of their immediate family. Some of those questions relate specifically to themselves and their prognosis, such as 'How long before I am in a wheelchair?' or 'Have I a severe or mild form of MS?', or even more starkly, 'How long have I got?'. Other questions relate more to their relationships to others, and particularly to implications for present or future families, such as 'Can I pass MS on to others – is it infectious?', or 'Should I marry?' and 'Should I have children?', or 'Will my children get MS?'. Such questions may exercise family members in as great a measure as those with the disease. Parents may wonder whether it is their fault that one of their children has the disease, spouses may wonder if the condition will be passed to them, children may wonder if they can acquire it from one of their parents.

Such expressions of concern are likely, especially with a condition with a mysterious aetiology and an uncertain prognosis. Seeking answers may be difficult where clinicians seem too busy or the questions too trivial to pose in the brisk atmosphere of a hospital or clinic. Patients and their families may take advantage of the often more relaxed contact with other professional staff, like physiotherapists, speech therapists, nurses, nutritionists or counsellors, to pose questions of a diverse and fundamental kind. For therapists such approaches may arise unexpectedly, and not be readily answerable from their own background and training.

The aim of this section of the chapter is to identify areas of concern which may arise when considering people and their families.

How early can the diagnosis be made?

From the perspective of a family in which one of its members may have a range of continuing and problematic symptoms, the question of when a formal clinical diagnosis can be made is a crucial one. As is noted in a more detailed discussion later in this chapter, major family decisions may depend on such knowledge.

As has been indicated in Chapter 2, there is no specific and certain laboratory test for the disease, and clinical diagnosis is contingent on an array of events occurring over time (Poser et al., 1983). There are laboratory tests which are used to support clinical diagnosis such as the measurement of visually evoked potential or the measurement of IgG levels in cerebrospinal fluid (Thompson et al., 1985) but none of the abnormalities thus demonstrated are specific to the disease. Attempts to produce specific blood tests for MS (Field, Joyce and Smith, 1977; Tamblyn et al., 1980; Jones et al., 1983) have met with only minimal success; however, research is continuing to seek to develop an effective test. The recent development of magnetic resonance imaging (MRI) has helped to produce more definitive pathological data on the condition (Paty et al., 1988). However, the procedure is expensive and access is confined to relatively few centres, and a positive MRI scan is not exclusive to MS (Sibley, 1988; p.6).

A recent report based on a 15-year follow-up of patients presenting with uncomplicated optic neuritis found that 74% of women and 34% of men went on to develop the disease within 15 years (Rizzo and Lessell, 1988). These authors further predict, on the basis of their study, that 20 years after presentation 91% of women and 44% of men may be expected to have developed MS. However, it is important to recognize the difficulties of directly extrapolating from initial findings in a condition such as MS. This study raises the question of whether patients and their families should be alerted to the possibility of optic neuritis being a harbinger of the disease,

155

particularly as in some research MRI scanning appears to reveal associated 'silent' cerebral lesions in a high proportion of cases (Ormerod *et al.*, 1986; Jacobs, Kinkel and Kinkel, 1986). The prediction of the onset of the disease on this basis must still be seen as one indicating possibility, rather than certainty.

In such a situation, where only broadly indicative laboratory tests are available and where clinical diagnosis is dependent on the temporal development of the condition, there is considerable latitude for different diagnostic practices, especially over the disclosure of the diagnosis to patients and their families. Some clinicians may reveal diagnoses at an early stage, others may delay the revelation for a considerable length of time for medical or managerial reasons. In the absence of scientifically validated and effective treatment clinicians may feel that disclosure can be delayed more than it would otherwise be. However, patients and their families may feel an inherent sense of frustration that something might have been done if knowledge, even of a possible diagnosis, had been gained earlier. The considerable consequences of some of these practices for families are discussed later in this chapter.

Is multiple sclerosis likely to infect my family or others?

In social and family situations the possibility of transmission of the disease from one person to another is often a matter of concern. Embedded in this concern is the supposition that the disease may be caused by an infectious or contagious agent. Drawing on present knowledge it is most unlikely that this supposition is correct.

During the chequered history of the search for the cause of MS a number of animal diseases which produce MS-like lesions or symptoms in particular animal species have been implicated as predisposing factors to humans developing MS. The most widely studied have been scrapie in sheep (Murrell, O'Donoghue and Ellis, 1986), distemper in dogs (Cook, Dowling and Russell, 1978; Kurtzke *et al.*, 1988). and a tick-borne infection *Borrelia burgdorferi*, often called Lyme disease (Schmutzhard, Pohl and Stanek, 1988).

In general, there is little formal support for the argument that MS is passed from animals to man by specific infectious agents, or passed in other ways, by blood transfusions for example. Further, any suggestions of this kind would have to take into account the differential susceptibility of individuals to the disease (considered in more detail below).

It follows that if an infectious agent in the genesis of MS is unlikely then familial, nursing or other intimate contact with someone with the condition, breast feeding for example, carries no risk of acquiring the disease.

Even if MS is unlikely to be infectious it still could conceivably be a condition with viral origins.

Is the disease caused by a virus?

Many lines of research suggest that a slow virus infection may be associated with the onset of MS. This suggestion has been derived from the observation that viral particles persist in the body fluids and central nervous system of people with the disease (Gunaddottir *et al.*, 1964). It is outside the scope of this book to review the many theories of viral involvement in MS. However, present opinion is largely that the disease is far more likely to be related to distur- bances in the immune system and the way that virus infections are managed in general by that system, rather than the presence of any specific virus itself. There is however evidence that relapses of MS may occur more frequently following common viral infections (Sibley, Bunford and Clark, 1985), and this argues for managerial strategies which minimize the risk of such infections by an appropriate diet and good health care.

How will the disease progress? Will I soon be in a wheelchair?

For families, predicting the future course of the disease is crucial to making decisions about many aspects of life. Unfortunately the capacity to predict the course of the disease is limited, both in the short and long term. A number of recent attempts have been made to evaluate possible predictive factors which might be of help, such as the extent of initial sensory or motor symptoms (Francis *et al.*, 1987), the age and sex of the patient concerned, and the pattern of relapses and remissions in the short term (Minderhoud, van der Hoeven and Prange, 1988). Using these and other factors, Compston (1987) has suggested that it may be possible to establish broad prognostic guidelines for certain categories of patients.

Other recent attempts to tackle the question of prognosis are based on the view that there are two categories into which the course of the disease may fall. One is characterized by an initial relapsing/remitting phase with the secondary development of a progressive phase, the other exhibits a progressive course from onset. Studies examining the first year during which the disease becomes progressive have yielded useful prognostic information (Minderhoud, van der Hoeven and Prange, 1988). The conclusion of this study shows that 63% of 342 patients were in the relapsing/remitting category, and of these 31% had already reached the secondary progressive phase. The remaining 37% of the patients showed a primary progressive course. However, the age at which the progressive phase of the disease appeared was similar at around 35 years. The authors conclude that disease progression is greatest in primary progressive disease, and thus the poorest prognosis is for those whose disease starts late and is immediately progressive – in which category there appear to be proportionately more males.

Despite this research the predictive power of the variables employed is still modest even for large groups of patients, let alone for individuals. There may be further possibilities for prognostic guidance as genetic indicators are systematically explored (see below). However, at present there is little that can be realistically indicated to individual patients and their families about the precise course of their own disease.

The issue of prognosis is especially apposite in relation to the search for effective therapies for MS. The balance between health problems caused by the unpredictably progressive condition, and those that may be caused by robust treatments designed to arrest it, is a major issue. Many of the available options for possible therapeutic efficacy in MS are based on the hypothesis that there is substantial immunological disturbance in relation to the disease. A range of immunosuppressive therapies are therefore being explored for their role in managing the condition. These immunosuppressive therapies are, for the most part, liable to produce side-effects of varying orders of severity if administered over a period of time (Kappos *et al.*, 1988). The difficulty is to balance the possible benefits of such therapies against their possible costs in terms of side-effects. This equation can only reliably be solved if precise prognostic indicators can be developed. For individuals and their families seeking to find ways of managing the condition themselves, a similar kind of dilemma exists. They will try and evaluate for themselves the costs involved in pursuing particular strategies, set against an estimation of the course and effects of the condition.

Thus prognostic understanding of MS is still in a relatively un-developed and imprecise state which makes the task of managing the condition difficult for both clinicians, and patients and their families.

To what extent is there a genetic factor in the disease? Is the disease inherited?

Perhaps the most frequently asked questions are those related to the risk of developing MS when other family members have the disease. The question raises complex issues, some aspects of which are more easily answered than others. It can be said that the disease is not genetically passed on to others in the same way as conditions such as haemophilia and muscular dystrophy where specific maternal genes, associated with the presence of certain paternal genes, combine to ensure a high risk of an affected child. MS is not a disease that is inherited in such a clear and unequivocal way. However, it is becoming recognized that increased susceptibility to many conditions such as heart disease, cancer and diabetes is related to genetic factors which are at present not well understood. In common with many other conditions, certain gene types appear to carry a susceptibility to develop the disease. It is important to recognize that this relationship only increases the possibility that MS will occur, it does not indicate that the disease is probable, and even less that it is inevitable.

Exactly which genetic groups are associated with an increased risk of developing MS is a matter of considerable debate. There is considerable research that has been undertaken in relation to this issue (Madigand *et al.*, 1982). The genetic marker usually associated with the disease is HLA (human lymphocyte antigen) DR2, which in most reports shows a frequency of about 60% in confirmed MS. Associations between the disease and an increased frequency of HLA A3 and B7 have also been noted (Batchelor, 1977).

However, research has not yet resulted in any clinically useful gene markers for MS. Further epidemiological studies of genetically or geographically isolated populations have, so far, only supported these observations for Caucasian groups, not for all those with MS (Brautbar, Amar and Cohen, 1982).

From the point of view of patients and their families the most helpful research at present is that which has assessed risks of the disease given certain familial relationships. The most recent evidence indicates that female members of a family in which the mother, an aunt or a sister have the disease carry an increased risk of developing it themselves, compared with situations where male family members are affected, or where there is no family history of the disease. This finding is not surprising in view of the fact that approximately twice the number of woman as men have the disease (Brunel-Arms Research Unit, 1983). More particularly first-order family members appear to have a 10 to 15% increased risk of developing the disease compared with people with no family history, whilst those with second or third-order relatives show only a 2 to 5% increased risk (Sadovnick and McLeod, 1981).

More complete risk assessment will only become available as the capacity to manipulate genetic material improves, and when the triggering or precipitating role of specific environmental factors on susceptibility to MS is better understood.

It can be seen from the above assessments in relation to scientific knowledge about the disease, its characteristics and risks that information in many areas is still incomplete. Broad guidance can be given on the basis of available knowledge. In many situations it is likely that patients and their families will not be satisfied with the uncertainties which remain in the advice which can legitimately be given. Thus these uncertainties will be added to and inform the way that family relationships and family dynamics develop with MS in their midst.

MULTIPLE SCLEROSIS AND FAMILY DYNAMICS

The experience of MS, as has been noted elsewhere in this book, may well be linked with disturbances in behaviour or states of mind. Uncertainty, anxieties about the past, present and future, and frustration with a declining body may all lead to changes in behaviour or attitudes (Grant, 1986). Families may respond to such situations in many different ways.

One way of managing a potentially damaging condition for both individuals and their families is to reject it, or aspects of it. Thoughts connected with the illness, or its associated symptoms or consequences may be denied in many different ways at different levels. It may be that the person with the disease will be completely rejected by their family; sometimes this occurs with the collusion of the person themselves as they feel that their family can only continue in a viable way if they leave it (Robinson, 1988a; Chapter 4).

A less complete rejection may also occur as the person with MS adopts attitudes and behaviours with considerable repercussions for others in social contact with them. In particular, patients may reject aspects of themselves which they consider lead to a problematic dependence on others, e.g. where they might be seen as having 'given in to MS'. This can leave such people fiercely fighting for independence but unable to seek, or to use, help realistically. On the other hand they may reject self-reliant aspects of themselves, becoming overtly and explicitly dependent on others, and denying the more negative feelings associated with being helped. Where either of these kinds of rejection take place they can substantially influence the behaviour of others, both informally amongst their family and more formally amongst those giving professional help.

There is substantial evidence that many patients with MS have adopted what might be described as a confrontational and aggressive approach to their condition, describing their actions as 'fighting MS' (Pollack, 1984). Indeed their personal survival is perceived as being contingent on these actions. Family members may or may not share such beliefs and their associated behaviours. Problems may arise through a patient's single-minded and constant pursuit of strategies which are deemed vital for individual well-being. In such cases the physical effects of the disease itself may be less difficult for a family to live with than managerial strategies which alter previous everyday understandings and expectations over behaviour and attitudes.

Part of the difficulty that families may have in this situation is in deciding whether to 'make allowances' for the bad or unusual behaviour of family members with MS. Such behaviour may be excused by reference to its assumed objectives, i.e. the search to control the condition, or by reference to the debilitating effects of the disease itself on the person's capacity to conform to the ordinary rules of family life (Power, 1985). However, relationships may fracture because each family member becomes embedded in their own problems. Their capacity to exercise reflective and benign judgements about others is lost in the preoccupation with their own difficulties. Family members without MS and the person with the disease may feel that the other is being unreasonably self-centred or selfish. A great deal of research and analysis (Bury, 1982; Charmaz, 1983) has demonstrated that there is a tendency for chronic illness to focus attention inward, rather than to facilitate acknowledgement of the claims of others for attention to their problems.

For some families a continual preoccupation by the person with the disease with their own problems can appear effectively to undermine or demolish the significance of the 'normal' problems of family living. In this process anger or bitterness may be expressed by family members about the withdrawal from involvement in such problems, and a corresponding resentment expressed by the person with MS that their point of view and difficulties are not understood (Cunningham, 1977).

On the other hand there may be a conflict between wanting to make allowances for those with MS, and not wanting to be patronizing. There is, however, a danger that 'making allowances' for someone with the disease may unhelpfully take away a central familial role by effectively excluding them from family decision making (Robinson, 1988b). In this respect people with MS may want special consideration at some times, and may get angry at other times if they are treated any differently from anyone else in the family.

In the complex social and personal world inhabited by people with MS and their families there may be major problems in discriminating between the direct and involuntary effects of the condition on behaviour and attitudes, and effects which may be voluntary and modifiable. Such a dilemma is summed up in the question, 'Is it him (or her), or is it the effects of MS?' Feelings of anger, withdrawal or preoccupation may be explained either way. A particularly problematic set of issues for family members occurs in relation to memory loss, confusion or other kinds of mental difficulty. Some such symptoms may be related to the disease state itself, others may be related to the presence of particular drug therapies, and yet others may be related to states of mind only indirectly or marginally contingent on the condition. Disentangling these possible pathways is a particular problem for family members.

Some cognitive and memory loss is not uncommon in the course of the disease (Grant et al., 1984). However, the ways in which such losses are manifest may be varied. A lack of ability to concentrate may occur; following and participating in discussions requiring a logical train of thought may be difficult; or forgetfulness may become part of the normal daily round of jobs and activities.

There are many ways of dealing with these mental and cognitive difficulties once they are recognized. However, their recognition may not only be problematic because losses may be gradual and incremental, but also because their very recognition is an acknowledgement of declining powers, and a changing sense of self-loss of these functions may be interpreted in ways which are frightening both to the person with the difficulties and to those with whom they live. For some people such a loss may mean losing their independence, or it may imply to them a loss of love or attention or the loss of their previous role in the family. It may imply a lessening of the ability to communicate their wishes and concerns, and perhaps above all it may imply a loss of control over themselves – especially for those who have made the mental fight against the disease a corner-stone of their lives.

One effect of the gradual loss of these abilities may be to lead to an increasing discrepancy between family members' perception of the capacities of the person with MS and their own perception. A number of studies have indicated that this is a common problem (Lincoln, 1981; Robinson, 1988b) with the person with the disease having a more positive perception of their capacities. This discrepancy in itself is likely to be associated with conflict. There may finally come the point where the person with MS is defined as incapable of making certain decisions.

Someone who has lost part of their mental capacity may feel strongly that something has been stolen from them. Family members may feel that in taking away decision-making power from a confused or mentally deteriorated member of the family, they are stealing the capacity of the person concerned, and also perhaps taking away their initiative at the same time. It may be very difficult to be sure whether their initiative has already gone as a result of damage to the central nervous system, or whether it only appears that this is the case because a family member has usurped decision making and prevented initiative from being taken.

HUSBANDS, WIVES AND PARTNERS

Multiple sclerosis often occurs when families are in the process of being formed, or adult relationships have recently been established. The coincidence of the disease with a major series of life stage developments means invariably that its effects, and perceptions of its nature, interlock with expectations about these relationships (Robinson, 1988a; Chapter 3). As many such relationships in early adulthood are potentially fragile it is never easy to distinguish the specific effects of the added presence of the disease from those problems which are endemically present in all partnerships. One of the dangers of a particular analysis of the role of MS is that its effects may be overemphasized, and the 'normal' difficulties which lead to casualties in partnerships or marriages underestimated.

Relationships, whether or not marriage is involved, have at their core visions and hopes for the future against which the potential constraints and problems posed by the disease must be set. As is noted elsewhere in this chapter it may be the case that problems crystallize around perceptions of the disease. MS may assume the role of a catalyst in bringing to the surface other conflicts and issues which might not otherwise seem so significant, in addition to its more specific impact through direct physical and mental deterioration.

Relationships may be discontinued once a diagnosis of MS is made known (Brooks and Matson, 1987). The uncertainty and possible effects of the condition thus precipitate a break in a relationship in which a further problem has been injected. Conversely there are those relationships which not only survive but flourish in the presence of the disease which seems to consolidate the partnership. Indeed, there are those who are brought together precisely because of the existence of the disease. It must not be thought therefore that MS has an entirely negative impact; as with most events and circumstances which transpire in the course of life it may be understood and acted upon in substantially different ways.

Nonetheless the continuation of a partnership with MS embedded in it is something which has to be seriously considered. It raises major questions about jobs and careers, about the ability to have and to rear children, and about the nature of the relationship in the future with more substantial disability associated with it (Miles, 1979). There are complex problems involved in all these areas which it is not possible to consider here in any detail.

Most relationships will survive in the setting of MS, but they may still be damaged in various ways. Some families appear to operate on the basis that only one partner can effectively be in control at the expense of the other. Where this happens they are unlikely to be able to care for each other without considerable friction, and they may even live apart but maintain contact at a distance. Thus it must not be assumed that all partners want what is best for each other. Selfishness, neglect and destructive behaviour can occur on both sides. One danger for the professional is becoming drawn into partisan involvement in such situations. This they should avoid, while trying to understand how to interpret and act on such problems effectively.

There may be related areas which raise difficulties for professional intervention. The frustration of having MS in a relationship may lead, with other factors, to the threat or actual use of physical violence. Many such incidents may not appear to be serious in their immediate effects; however they are indicative of a serious malaise in a relationship. For the most part such matters are rarely directly reported outside the relationship, either for fear that dramatic action may be taken, or more probably in the realization that the information will not be taken seriously. From a therapist's point of view it may take courage to explore this area and referral to specialist help may well be required. In the hidden agenda of family life which may be exposed through professional contact, clues indicating such problems should be pursued, always with the help of experienced colleagues or others.

Whilst this section has indicated a range of problems often associated with the presence of MS, it must be recognized that family relationships are of many different kinds. The temptation may be to assume that the family structure of patients and their relationships are similar to those of the therapists who are treating them. The indications are that the range of relationships amongst people with MS, their marriages and their partnerships, are as complex and multifaceted as amongst those without the disease.

WILL BECOMING PREGNANT MAKE MY MULTIPLE SCLEROSIS WORSE?

Understanding of the impact of pregnancy on the course of multiple sclerosis by clinicians and medical researchers has changed substantially over recent years. On the basis of unsystematic clinical observation medical opinion was formerly that pregnancy constituted a grave risk for women with multiple sclerosis, indeed '. . . it was regarded as an important indication for termination . . .' (Matthews *et al.*, 1985; p.85). Cumulative scientific research on the relationship between pregnancy and the disease has now produced a very different picture. The major and relatively consistent finding of this research has been that pregnancy itself, particularly in the first two trimesters, is associated with a lower rate than expected of relapses of the disease in those women with a non-progressive form of multiple sclerosis (Birk and Rudick, 1986). On the other hand the rate of relapses in the postpartum period, particularly in the first three months postpartum, is substantially greater amongst such women than would normally be anticipated (Nelson, Franklin and Jones, 1988). However, the interpretation of these findings is not easy particularly if a longer-term view is taken.

There is little evidence that women who have been pregnant experience more relapses overall than other women. This is so even

165

in a comparison of a 15-month period including the pregnancy and six months postpartum (Frith and McLeod, 1988). Reinforcing this point in another way, an earlier study found no difference after a set duration of the disease between women who had been pregnant and those who had not (Poser *et al.*, 1979). Indeed, in one recent but, it should be said, unsupported study following patients over a 25-year period in Sweden, women with the disease who had had pregnancies appeared to have a better longer-term prognosis than other women (Runmarker and Anderson, 1989). It may be the case that pregnancy precipitates or 'anticipates' relapses that would otherwise happen later, or that the sequencing of relapses is different in pregnant women. In either case there is little formal evidence to support the negative view that used to be commonly taken by medical advisors. Breast feeding appears not be associated with any different path of the disease (Nelson, Franklin and Jones, 1988). As long as the increased risk of immediate post-partum relapse is acknowledged, and as much care is taken as possible in the management of the condition, there appears to be no general reason why pregnancy should not be undertaken by women with multiple sclerosis.

It should be said that many of the previously negative attitudes towards pregnancy of women with the disease appeared to stem as much from concern about the role of mothers with disabilities managing their children, as from the particular effects of the disease itself (National Childbirth Trust, 1984). As attitudes change towards such women a more positive attitude should manifest itself amongst both medical practitioners and the population at large.

PARENTS AND CHILDREN

The relationship between parents and children is of particular importance in MS. This is not only because the disease may well occur at a time when decisions have to be made about the possibility of having children, but also at a time when their upbringing and socialization is of major concern. Some of these children may themselves become involved in a specifically caring role for a parent or other family member at an early age, or feel responsible for the care of a parent with the disease later in life. On the other hand there will be many situations where older parents have children affected by the disease in early adulthood. In each of these situations there are likely to be particular issues and problems which arise

166

influencing the nature and outcome of family relationships (Cunningham, 1977).

Older parents with children affected in early adulthood face a range of issues. They may be faced with a major reorientation of their expectations over the future of their child, and perhaps also be faced with unexpected practical consequences at a time when direct family responsibilities for children are usually declining. In this situation some parents may find that they have been given a new and clear role in life as a carer. However, continuation of the maternal role may be welcome to some, if problematic for others. Amongst this latter group are those looking forward to a life of their own, as well as those who may have physical problems or disabilities themselves. Such a situation may also complicate the relationship between the parents themselves. However, feelings are rarely simple, and attitudes of resentment towards this new situation may be accompanied by concern and anxiety for the future of the child, as well as a strong wish to do everything possible to help. Mothers, and perhaps fathers, may blame themselves for the illness.

Parents may also be concerned as to what is going to happen to their child when they can no longer look after him, or when they are dead. Thinking about residential care may seem disloyal, or even considering it may appear to hasten the time when it is necessary.

Children with MS may also have ambivalent attitudes about the renewed parental attention which is visited on them at a point when they would have normally sought further independence from parental control. On the one hand they may feel grateful for the support which is available from this quarter in a future which has been concertinaed into the present; on the other hand, to be catapulted backwards into a more dependent role may merely serve to exacerbate their feelings of loss of self reliance. In this latter group parents may be seen by either their affected son or daughter, or by others, as being overprotective. In either case the relationship between parent and child is not likely to be easily dealt with. From the point of view of professional intervention, negotiations with parents and children in this situation may be especially difficult, with radically different expectations as to who has, or should have, control of the family management of the condition.

Where a parent is affected him- or herself there may be a series of problems which arise in their relationships with their children. Some of these are to do with their perception of their family role: whether they can be a 'proper' father or mother and whether they can be fully involved in the upbringing of children, or indeed whether they are being totally marginalized in the management of their family relationships. They may fear unfavourable comparisons by their children between their 'disabled' state, and that of the un-affected parent or other adults of the same sex. Perhaps as a result of these problems there may be a tendency to overcompensate in terms of the control or disciplining of family life, a practice which may compound the issues which resulted in the overcompensation in the first place. An affected parent's family role is therefore a difficult one to establish with security, not least because it is likely that the increasing physical prowess of children as they grow older will be mirrored by a corresponding physical decline of the parent. It is hard to be detached from this striking and unequal physical equation.

For young or adolescent children with affected parents there are special sets of difficulties which up until recently have been largely unrecognized. The lack of a clear source of professional help for them and an insulated family environment may make their lives particularly hard. They may not be able to tell their parents their most painful anxieties about their parents' or their own deaths, or about their fears of their role in causing the disease or about whether they can catch the disease. They may not be able to discuss their own identification with disability which may undermine their self-confidence, or their fears of being left with the sole responsibility for the care of their parent. They may also be acting in a caring role for their affected parent, performing intimate tasks of body maintenance. This role and these tasks may not only be tiring and continuous but may also in effect run the risk of undermining their own growth to independence through adolescence, or may project them too quickly through childhood to premature adult roles.

Nurses, doctors, social workers and others may all be in a position to listen carefully to the problems of such children and any anxieties and concerns, both practical and emotional, they may have.

PROFESSIONAL INVOLVEMENT WITH FAMILIES

Uncertainty in dealing with the consequences of MS and its manage-ment permeates the relationship of the professional with the patient and his/her family as it does the day-to-day lives of patients themselves. Knowledge and information seem to offer some sense of control, but as has already been indicated, there remain many scien-tific and medical uncertainties in relation to the condition. Therefore therapists may find that it is difficult to meet the expectations of patients and their families, and find themselves in situations where their interactions are complex and problematic.

It may be tempting in such situations to consider patients with MS and their families as especially difficult, or as 'problem families'. Whether there really are more 'problem families' with MS than without the disease is difficult to prove. The issue hinges on definitions of what constitutes the 'problem'. For families themselves difficulties may reside in, and be exacerbated by, the professionals they meet. However, there are certainly families whose members appear to present major managerial difficulties to a range of professional staff.

It appears that at times the symptoms of MS may undermine peoples' maturity, and allow or encourage them to regress temporarily to a more childlike state. An array of symptoms associated with a different life stage, such as incontinence, an inability to feed oneself independently or be mobile, may precipitate reactions of a kind which makes professional intervention difficult.

At such times people with MS may feel more persecuted or less able to use words to convey information and may substitute behaviour to convey experiences. They may feel that the choices are stark and categorical, rather than continuous and incremental, and they may fear situations that are relatively uncontrollable. The remaining family members may find that this change is difficult to understand, and the loss of reasonableness on the patient's part, albeit temporarily, reflects their own concerns about the uncertain and unpredictable future.

It may also be the case that a patient or a member of their family conflates their experience with MS with that of other damaging personal experiences in their lives, for example with unloving or untrustworthy parents. In this situation the therapist or the doctor may become another extension of a particularly traumatic relationship, in which there is a lack of trust in both the judgement and the objectives of the professional concerned. It can be the case that patients or a member of their families manage the therapist–client relationship in such a way that this expectation becomes true.

On the other hand there are also situations where professional incompetence, or lack of concern, is indeed manifest without the collusion of the patient or their family. The fact that professionals sometimes fail to take actions that they have indicated they would, or behave in ways which are arguably not in the patient's interest, may reinforce these suspicions and concerns. In a situation such as that presented by MS where patients may expect continuing relationships with professional staff over long periods of time, relatively short-term contact for specific therapeutic purposes may be treated as further evidence of professional disinterest in the patient's longer-term problems and goals. Therefore, the consequences of professional judgement and the limitations of available resources may substantively conflict with what family members, as well as the patient, expect from formal health care.

Professional staff may need to tolerate uncomfortable feelings in being perceived by the patient or their family as not providing what is necessary. Going beyond the immediate difficulties caused by such feelings to an understanding of their possible sources in the patient's own earlier life, or their previous professional contacts, can deepen the therapist–client relationship. However not all professional staff may be willing or able to take such a view, and in this situation referral to counsellors or psychotherapists may be more appropriate.

Differences in family structure and functioning may be clearly related to the ability of the therapist to work with patients. There are many different kinds of families, some of which are more personally rewarding to work with than others. Those families which appear to demonstrate a high level of care for each other, whilst on the other hand acknowledging their individual differences and aspirations, repay professional time spent with them. They appear to take what is professionally offered and add it to their own enthusiasm and abilities in a profitable partnership. Mutual respect is easier to maintain, dependence is not dreaded, despair is temporary and bearable, and anxieties can be shared with others and reduced.

Other family structures are not of this kind and appear to involve, perhaps even depend on, the existence of confrontation, anger or bitterness which is reflected both internally in relationships inside the family, and externally in relationships with professional staff. Such effects in a family with MS may help to create the picture that some professionals describe, of people with the disease, and their families, being particularly difficult. However, it is important to recognize that the disease may also arouse fears and feelings in therapists and others professionally dealing with such people and their families, whose own personal actions and behaviour may be affected, whatever formal training they may have had in distancing themselves from such personal involvement.

There are significant consequences for families inviting or allowing professional interventions. A good experience may not only allow such interventions to improve quality of life with the disease, but may encourage other helpful contacts, whereas an unsuccessful encounter may not only deprive the patient and the family of immediate assistance, but also inhibit or actually prevent future requests for help.

Many therapeutic interventions need the support of the family to be effectively undertaken, but that support cannot be assumed. The process of bringing a patient into hospital may be costly in terms of time, resources or goodwill, and families may feel that asking for help, and undertaking the necessary steps to accomplish access to it, require major changes in their personal or family situation. Appointments for therapy may result in significant alterations in both the practical and emotional aspects of daily family life, and professionals need to be aware of this and make every effort to ensure that appointments are kept at the time stated, and that where delays occur the legitimacy of patients', or their families', distress or anger is acknowledged.

Families of people with MS are likely to be substantially involved in therapeutic strategies for the management of the disease, and they anticipate professional concern about their role as well as professional guidance and support (Simons, 1984).

CONCLUSION

Families are essentially complex structures. The interplay of the needs and expectations of individuals, combined with the working of the family as a whole, produces a wide range of attitudes and patterns of behaviour, many of which are difficult to interpret easily from the outside. The addition of chronic illness in this situation, in the form of MS, compounds these complexities. The normal uncertainties of life will be increased, existing conflicts and problems may be exacerbated, and other latent difficulties become evident. Thus family members, including any with MS, are not just dealing with the condition alone, but are managing it in the context of all aspects of their lives.

In this situation hard information about the physical effects and consequences of the condition is highly significant. However, much information about the disease is not categorical or certain, and invariably it will be filtered through the prism of existing family relationships. Similarly therapeutic actions will be considered by patients and their families, not just for their physical consequences, whether they be dramatic and positive, marginal or negative, but for the ways in which they contribute to the personal or familial goals at a more general level. For this reason it is important for professional staff to acknowledge that although they may see their particular role as specific and targeted towards discrete and measurable effects, they are working in an environment where their clients and their families may have quite different ideas and objectives. The reconciliation of the objectives of clients, their families and the therapists involved should thus be a major concern of good professional practice, and may be essential for the proper operation of that practice.

REFERENCES

Batchelor, J.R. (1987) Histocompatibility antigens and their relevance to multiple sclerosis. *British Medical Bulletin,* **19**, 72–5.

Birk, H. and Rudick, R. (1986) Pregnancy and multiple sclerosis. *Archives of Neurology,* **43**, 719–26.

Brautbar, C., Amar, A. and Cohen, N. (1982) HLA-D typing in MS: Israelis tested with European homozygous typing cells. *Tissue Antigens* **19**, 89–197.

Brooks, N. and Matson, R.R. (1987) Managing multiple sclerosis, in *The Experience and Management of Chronic Illness* (eds J.A. Roth and P. Conrad). JAI Press, Greenwich, Conn., pp. 73–106.

Brunel-ARMS Research Unit (1983) More Women than Men? Questioning the Facts. Academic Working Paper. Brunel-Arms Research Unit, Dept. of Human Sciences, Brunel University, West London.

Burnfield, A. (1985) *Multiple Sclerosis: A personal exploration.* Souvenir Press, London.

Bury, M. (1982) Chronic illness as biographical disruption. *Sociology of Health and Illness,* **4**, 167–82.

Charmaz, K. (1983) Loss of self: a fundamental form of suffering in the chronically ill. *Sociology of Health and Illness,* **5**, 168–95.

Compston, A. (1987) Can the course of MS be predicted, in *More Dilemmas in the Management of the Neurological Patient* (eds C. Warlow and J. Garfield). Churchill Livingstone, Edinburgh, pp. 45–50.

Cook, S.D., Dowling, P.C. and Russell, W.C. (1978) Multiple sclerosis and canine distemper. *Lancet,* **i**, 605–6.

Cunningham, D.J. (1977) Stigma and Social Isolation: Self Perceived Problems of a Group of Multiple Sclerosis Sufferers. Report No.27, Health Services Research Unit, Centre for Research in the Social Sciences, University of Kent, Canterbury.

Field, E.J., Joyce, G. and Smith, B.M. (1977) Erythrocyte-UFA (Eufa) mobility tests for multiple sclerosis: implications for pathogenesis and handling of the disease. *Journal of Neurology,* **214**, 113–27.

Francis, D.A., Compston, D.S.A., Batchelor, J.R. *et al.* (1987) A reassessment of the risk of multiple sclerosis developing in patients with optic neuritis after extended follow-up. *Journal of Neurology, Neurosurgery and Psychiatry,* **50**, 758–65.

Frith, J.A. and McLeod, J.G. (1988) Pregnancy and multiple sclerosis. *Journal of Neurology, Neurosurgery and Psychiatry*, **51**, 495–8.

Grant, I. (1986) Neuropsychological and psychiatric disturbances in multiple sclerosis, in *Multiple Sclerosis* (eds W.I. McDonald and D.H. Silberberg). Butterworth, London.

Grant, I., McDonald, W.I., Trimble, M.R. *et al.* (1984) Deficient learning and memory in early and middle phases of multiple sclerosis. *Journal of Neurology, Neurosurgery and Psychiatry*, **47**, 250–5.

Gunaddottir, M., Helgadottir, H., Bjarnason, O. *et al.* (1964) Virus isolated from the brain of patients with multiple sclerosis. *Experimental Neurology*, **9**, 85–95.

Jacobs, L., Kinkel, P.R. and Kinkel, W.R. (1986) Silent brain lesions in patients with optic neuritis: a clinical and nuclear magnetic resonance imaging study. *Archives of Neurology*, **43**, 495–511.

Jones, R., Preece, A.W., Luckman, N.P., *et al.* (1983) The analysis of the red cell unsaturated fatty acid test for multiple sclerosis using laser cytopherometry. *Physics in Medicine and Biology*, **28**, 1145–51.

Kappos, L., Patzold, U., Dommasch, D. *et al.* (1988) Cyclosporine versus azathioprine in the long-term treatment of multiple sclerosis – results of the German multi centre study. *Annals of Neurology*, **23**, 56–63.

Kurtzke, J.F., Hyllested, K., Arbuckle, J.D. *et al.* (1988) Multiple sclerosis in the Faroe Islands. IV: the lack of a relationship between canine distemper and epidemics of MS. *Acta Neurologica Scandinavica*, **78**, 484–500.

Lincoln, N.B. (1981) Discrepancies between capabilities and performance of activities of daily living in multiple sclerosis patients. *International Rehabilitation Medicine*, **3**, 84–8.

Madigand, M., Oger, F.J.F., Fauchet, R. *et al.* (1982) HLA profiles in multiple sclerosis suggest two forms of disease and the existence of protective halotypes. *Journal of Neurological Science*, **53**, 519–29.

Matthews, W.B., Acheson, E.D., Batchelor, J.R. *et al.* (1985) *McAlpine's Multiple Sclerosis*. Churchill Livingstone, London.

Miles, A. (1979) Some psycho-social consequences of multiple sclerosis: problems of physical interaction and group identity. *British Journal of Medical Psychology*, **52**, 321–31.

Minderhoud, J.M., van der Hoeven, J.H. and Prange, A.J.A. (1988) Course and prognosis of chronic progressive multiple sclerosis. *Acta Neurologica Scandinavica*, **78**, 10–15.

Murrell, T.G.C., O'Donoghue, P.J. and Ellis, T. (1986) A review of the sheep–multiple sclerosis connection. *Medical Hypotheses*, **19**, 27–39.

National Childbirth Trust (1984) *The Emotions and Experiences of Disabled Mothers*. National Childbirth Trust, London.

Nelson, N.M., Franklin, G.M. and Jones, M.C. (1988) Risk of multiple sclerosis exacerbation during pregnancy and breast feeding. *Journal of the American Medical Association*, **259**, 3441–3.

Ormerod, I., McDonald, W.I., duBoulay, G.H. *et al.* (1986) Disseminated lesions at presentation with optic neuritis. *Journal of Neurology, Neurosurgery and Psychiatry*, **49**, 124–7.

Paty, D.W., Oger, F.J.F., Kastrukoff, L.F. *et al.* (1988) MRI in the diagnosis of MS: a prospective study with comparison of clinical evaluation, evoked potentials, oligoclonal banding and CT. *Neurology*, **38**, 180–5.

Pollack, K. (1984) Mind and Matter. Ph.D. thesis, Cambridge University.

Poser, C.M., Paty, D.W., Scheinberg, L.C. *et al.* (1983) New diagnostic criteria for multiple sclerosis: guidelines for research protocols. *Annals of Neurology,* **13**, 227–31.

Poser, S., Raun, N.E., Wikstrom, J. *et al.* (1979) Pregnancy, oral contraceptives and multiple sclerosis. *Acta Neurologica Scandinavica,* **55**, 108–18.

Power, P.W. (1985) Family coping behaviours in chronic illness: a rehabilitation perspective. *Rehabilitation Literature,* **46**, 78–83.

Rizzo, J.F. and Lessell, S. (1988) Risk of developing multiple sclerosis after uncomplicated optic neuritis: a long-term prospective study. *Neurology,* **38**, 185–90.

Robinson, I. (1988a) *Multiple Sclerosis.* Tavistock Publications, London.

Robinson, I. (1988b) Reconstructing lives: living with multiple sclerosis, in *Living with Chronic Illness* (eds R. Anderson and M. Bury). Unwin Hyman, London.

Runmarker, B. and Anderson, O. (1989) Prognostic factors in multiple sclerosis incidence material at a 25 year follow up, in *Recent Advances in Multiple Sclerosis Therapy* (eds R.E. Gonsette and P. Delmotte) Excepta Medica, Amsterdam, pp. 23–6.

Sadovnick, A.D. and McLeod, P.M.J. (1981) The familial nature of multiple sclerosis: risks for 1st, 2nd and 3rd degree relatives of patients. *Neurology,* **31**, 1039–41.

Schmutzhard, E., Pohl, P. and Stanek, G. (1988) *Borrelia burgdorferi* antibodies in patients with relapsing/remitting form and chronic progressive form of multiple sclerosis. *Journal of Neurology, Neurosurgery and Psychiatry,* **51**, 1215–18.

Sibley, W.A. (1988) *Therapeutic Claims in Multiple Sclerosis,* 2nd edn. Macmillan Press, London.

Sibley, W.A., Bunford, C.R. and Clark, K. (1985) Clinical virus infections and multiple sclerosis. *Lancet,* **i**, 131.

Simons, A. (1984) Problems of providing support for people with multiple sclerosis and their families, in *Multiple Sclerosis: Psychological and Social Aspects* (ed. A. Simons). Heinemann Medical, London.

Tamblyn, C.H., Swank, R.L., Seaman, G.V.F. *et al.* (1980) Red cell electrophoretic mobility test for early diagnosis of multiple sclerosis. *Neurological Research,* **2**, 69–83.

Thompson, A.J., Hutchinson, M., Martin, E.A. *et al.* (1985) Suspected and clinically definite multiple sclerosis: the relationship between CSF immunoglobulins and clinical course. *Journal of Neurology, Neurosurgery and Psychiatry,* **48**, 989–94.

FURTHER READING

Forti, A.D. and Segal, J. (1987) *MS and Pregnancy.* ARMS (Action and Research for Multiple Sclerosis) Publication, Stansted, Essex.

Koch-Hemiksen, N. (1990) An epidemiological study of multiple sclerosis: familial aggregation, social determinants and exogenic factors. *Acta Neurologica Scandinavica,* **80**, supplement 124.

12

When has therapy succeeded, and for whom?

Jennifer Worthington

Diseases that are characterized by a pattern of fluctuating symptoms or periods of relapse and recovery present a number of problems to the investigator wishing to evaluate the effects of a particular treatment. Multiple sclerosis (MS) is such a disease, with an unpredictable and progressive course. Because it is also a disease with an unknown aetiology and without a specific treatment, more remedies have been proposed for MS than almost any other condition. Today there are many anti-inflammatory, immuno-suppressive and anti-viral agents currently undergoing clinical trials but at least 120 other treatment for MS have been proposed over the years (Waksman, 1983). These approaches to treatment have changed over the years since the disease was first described in 1822, but many have not been evaluated clearly, if at all. Thus, there is a need for precise and carefully considered evaluation of treatments and therapies.

Because of the difficulties of assessing the efficacy of any treatment in a disease like MS, results from trials are often confusing for both the medical profession and for the patient. From this vast array of therapies doctors will often choose the most accepted treatments for the patient. Therapists will often choose the approaches to treatment they are skilful at rather than new treatment proposed in the literature, as 'therapy' is often more difficult to evaluate than a new drug. And how do patients decide which treatments are useful? MS is a life-long experience and as symptoms change and function is lost people's needs change. Patients are always making decisions about treatment, but trial results and advice from medical professionals are only one aspect in their decision-making process. The patient's evaluation of whether a treatment is successful or not may not be based on the same criteria that the medical profession would use.

The difficulties in evaluating the efficacy of treatment in MS are numerous. Level of symptoms can fluctuate daily and the patient will perform better when assessed on a 'good day'. It then becomes difficult to decide if the improvement is the result of treatment or a fluctuation in symptoms. Relapses and remissions occur with no set pattern and it is very difficult to delineate the end of a relapse clearly. If treatments are evaluated during this transition period misleading conclusions can be drawn. Evaluation techniques must be clearly defined and consistent even to begin to overcome these difficulties. There are a number of guidelines for research protocols involving MS patients (Weiner and Ellison, 1983; Poser, *et al.*, 1984) which address some of the difficulties in assessing treatments for this disease.

Evaluation must be carried out for a particular purpose and the first stage must be clearly to define the problem and the exact nature of the evaluative process. If this is not done it may be difficult to draw conclusions from any results. Evaluation is also carried out for a particular audience and thus the reason for evaluating a particular problem in the first place must be clear. Possible reasons might be to improve service to a particular group of patients in a therapist's or doctor's care, to alleviate a particular symptom for patients in general, to convince funding bodies that a service or treatment is worthwhile, to decide between competing usages of resources or to persuade patients to continue with therapy.

Other areas need defining. Success means different things to different people, but it can only be measured against the initial goals. This is particularly important in relation to treatments for MS, as what the researcher has succeeded in doing may not be the success the therapist or the patient wanted. Also, if the level of success is not clearly stated in the conclusions, the treatment may be used in inappropriate ways and then fail for both the therapist and the patient, or in repeated trials.

It is, however, more difficult to define the treatment. On one level, treatments can be quantified as to the amount given, for example, the quantity of a drug or the hours spent in physiotherapy. However, treatment is never as simple as this. The effect of a drug on a measurable physiological function is fairly straightforward but the results in this situation are only applicable to the tested function and tell us nothing about the success of the treatment. What is actually being evaluated is often difficult to define or to quantify. Treatment also encompasses the doctor/therapist/patient relationship and psychological/emotional reactions to treatment. Defining what constitutes therapy is often more elusive. Therapy must be flexible, responding to the daily needs of the patient. Therapy requires more contact hours than the administration of a drug, and therefore the aspects described above may need to be seen as part of the treatment process.

Once the evaluation of a treatment is completed, and if successful from the point of view of the researcher, consideration should be given to whether or not the treatment has also been successful for the patient. Important criteria from the patient's point of view might be the magnitude of the improvement, cost, energy and time spent travelling to and from the treatment. Conversely, an unsuccessful treatment from the researcher's point of view may be seen as worthwhile by the patient because it has indirectly alleviated a symptom or provided for the patient a better way of managing a symptom.

Once the problem to be studied has been clearly defined and thought has been given to the issues mentioned above, the therapy or treatment can be evaluated. This process should consider both the objective medical response and the patient's own view. The intention of this chapter is not to cover all aspects of this process, but to discuss several relevant questions. If it is assumed that there will be a change following a treatment, what are the goals of treatment, how is the change to be evaluated, how many people must show the same change, and is the change relevant to the patient and his/her life style?

WHAT ARE THE GOALS OF TREATMENT?

For MS, a disease with a progressive course, perhaps interspersed with relapses and periods of remission, improving clinical status may not be the most appropriate goal of treatment. Weiner and Ellison (1983) describe four goals that would be relevant for evaluating treatment in MS: 1) modify an ongoing exacerbation; 2) halt disease progression; 3) decrease frequency and severity of further relapses, and 4) improve the level of neurologic function in the clinically stable patient. Other goals could include improvement in symptom management and functional ability.

If the goal of treatment is slowing of disease progression or decreased relapse rate the effects of treatment need to be followed long term. For MS these treatments may be necessary throughout a patient's life and this has implications for patient compliance. This is especially true where the treatment is not going to halt the disease but may only alter its course.

Long-term treatments, such as diet, must be undertaken outside the hospital setting and require motivation from the patient. It is

177

important here clearly to identify for the patient what the treatment will and will not accomplish. A clear understanding of how treatment may be affecting the disease is necessary. Follow-up, then, must also be long term to determine if such treatments have an effect over time on the course of the disease.

Long-term use of medication may also be necessary, both for symptom management and alteration of the course of the disease. Compliance with taking medication appears to involve more than simply remembering to take the tablet. Conrad (1985) examined what medication meant to a group of 80 patients with epilepsy, and found that self-regulation of medication is one way for patients to gain some control over their condition. Reasons patients gave for reducing or discontinuing medication were to avoid unwanted side-effects that hindered daily social affairs, to check for progression or stabilization of the disorder, to feel less dependent on the medication and to avoid stagmatization. Patients would also increase their medication at times of stressful situations. These issues can affect both a research trial and results in a clinical setting.

If the goal of treatment is improvement in the level of neurologic function or in a specific parameter this should be clearly defined. In addition, the magnitude of the expected change and how long the improvement can be maintained is important. For example, if all patients in a treatment group show a small improvement with 'treatment A', but not 'B', this change is likely to be statistically significant. However, this small change may not be of any use in the clinical setting as the parameter being measured may still be in the abnormal range and have no noticeable effect on the patient's everyday life. In other words, statistical significance is not the same as clinical significance.

On the other hand, it may be that a small change is of benefit to one patient but not another. Individual social and personal factors can become important in determining the efficacy of a treatment. A small improvement in lower limb movements may be enough to delay the use of a wheelchair for a patient who is able to walk, but may be of no benefit to someone already using a wheelchair. Treatments that improve a symptom marginally, such as in bladder function, may not be considered successful by the researcher but may be highly significant for the patient. Thus, a treatment may be clinically significant but not statistically significant.

Physiotherapy and treatments that improve symptom management can result in improved ability in functional or daily activities. Even though there is no change in the course of the disease, functional gains improve the quality of life and are significant to the patient.

One also needs to consider whether improvements following a new treatment could be due to a placebo response. New treatments and participation in research trials often produce high expectation and increased motivation on the part of the patient. As mentioned above, this is particularly important when using performance measures as part of the assessment procedure. Worthington *et al.* (1987) found walking times significantly improved in the placebo group of an HBO trial, and this improvement was maintained until the end of the 4-month trial period. As walking is a performance-related test improved confidence or high motivation could produce such a result. However, a placebo response does not usually last for months. It is more likely that in a motivated group this improved functional ability could be due to the utilization of 'reserves' in the neuromuscular system.

Perhaps these functional gains that are maintained in a placebo group should be considered valid improvements, as they would certainly improve the quality of life when viewed from the patient's point of view. It may be, then, that treatments are more successful for the motivated patient. If so, then these encouraging aspects need to be considered as part of the treatment.

CAN THIS CHANGE BE EVALUATED?

In MS there is no readily available test of disease activity (MRI scanning may prove to be one in the future) and as a result there are a variety of tests and assessments that may be appropriate, depending on the question to be studied. Assessment, then, implies measurement, usually of some physical, mental or sensory response of the patient. That which is not measurable and quantifiable is often not taken into account. Assessment tools must be valid, that is, they have been shown to measure what they are supposed to measure. Assessment conditions should be consistent, both in setting and over time. In addition, baseline measurements on several occasions are valuable. This is especially true in a fluctuating disease such as MS. Assessment is usually classified as objective or subjective. Subjective assessment is based on the patient's evaluation of their symptoms and changes that occur with treatment, while objective measures are those made by the examiner.

There are a variety of questionnaires and subjective health measures available, such as the Nottingham Health Profile (McEwen, 1983). These are based on patient reports and can both quantify changes in health and also the effects of these changes on daily life. In addition methods exist to analyse qualitative data, such as that from interviews. A more complete discussion of the use of subjective data has been written by McDowell and Nevell (1987).

Objective tests fall into two categories. Some tests measure a quantifiable function where the answer is independent of the examiner's judgement, such as blood tests. These can only measure one function, but can monitor fine changes. These measures, although more repeatable and more definable, can only tell us something about the specific function being measured and not about the effect of treatment on the whole person.

Other tests rely on the examiner's ability to judge where on a scale a particular function lies, such as scales of grading muscle power. The most reliable scales are yes/no choices with only two points rather than a range of possible scores. These tests rely on observation and judgement. However, these measures give a better picture of overall functional ability of the patient and a better idea of disease status. On the other hand, the scales of measurement used here tend to be gross, with only marked changes in symptoms or functional abilities being reflected in a change of score. Finer improvements perceived by the patient, such as improved ability to pick up a cup, may not be seen on such assessments. It is also important to remember that these are often performance measures which require patient motivation. Patients can often perform better when re-tested for a variety of reasons, such as familiarity with the test, increased motivation because of the new treatment, or simply trying to better their previous performance.

Researchers often tend to give more weight to objective measures rather than subjective ones, arguing that changes must be measurable, and that objectivity implies accuracy and lack of bias. However, almost all forms of measurement carry some bias and room for error. Physiological measures require both skill of the operator at performing the test, such as an electromyogram, or some level of concentration on the part of the patient, such as a Visual Evoked Response test. Tests which rely on observation of a particular functional ability are dependent on the evaluator's ability to make consistent judgements and a consistent level of motivation from the patient. These are both considered to be objective tests. Thus, when objective tests are viewed from this perspective their relation to subjective measures can be seen as overlapping.

Patient reports often tend to contradict the findings of objective tests. Patients often perceive themselves as better for a variety of reasons and the improvement may not be apparent to the examiner. During a recent HBO trial (Worthington *et al.*, 1987), one participant listed urinary frequency as one of her symptoms which was confirmed by a 3-day urinary frequency chart. At the end of the trial this participant felt that bladder function was greatly improved, but her corresponding 3-day frequency chart showed no change in urinary frequency from pre-trial levels. It later emerged that during her participation in the trial her housing difficulties had been resolved and her toilet was now more accessible.

Clearly, decisions must be made about whose opinion, the examiner's or the patient's, is to be regarded as more valid. If both are to be used thought must be given to dealing with discrepancies. In the case above, the examiner could find no objective change in bladder function, while the patient felt that she had improved. Who is right? If the subjective findings are stated more clearly, e.g. the patient's perception of the severity of her symptoms had changed and her bladder function was no longer perceived to be as disabling as it was pre-trial, then this is a valid opinion that is relevant to the patient's everyday life. The fact that it was not a change observed by the examiner or that it quite likely had nothing to do with the treatment under evaluation is probably also irrelevant to the patient. For these reasons objective and subjective findings often show discrepancies, mainly because the subjective findings are not appropriately analysed.

Tests and assessment tools chosen should be relevant to the question to be studied and meaningful to the audience who will be interested in the study. Even though some assessments are more objective than others, these should not be the only criteria with which to choose. It would seem, then, that a mixture of objective and subjective measures would give us a better idea of the effect of a treatment.

HOW MANY PEOPLE MUST SHOW THE SAME CHANGE?

Traditionally in MS treatments are tested using a group comparison approach, and quite often the double-blind controlled trial. In order for a clinical trial to be considered valid and comparable to other similar trials certain rules must be rigidly applied. Weiner and Ellison (1983), in their guidelines for trials involving MS patients, have described disease categories, inclusion and exclusion criteria, sample size, etc. These considerations can become very cumbersome when dealing with MS because of the great variability among patients. In the clinical trial the sample size must be large enough to account for this variability and for the amount of benefit that the treatment being evaluated is expected to produce. In other words, large numbers may be necessary when evaluating a treatment on a group of relapse–remitting patients rather than stable MS patients. Similarly, a treatment that is expected to show a small benefit rather than a major one requires large numbers. With control groups of equal size, trials can easily require 100–200 participants, large numbers are often difficult to obtain and trials can become very lengthy or involve more than one centre. Another requirement of the clinical trial is random sampling. In practice this is difficult. A random sample of MS patients must adequately represent the various symptoms of the disease. However, patients available for trial participation often do not fit into the required categories. Some characteristics will be over-represented while others may not be adequately sampled. When randomly assigned to treatment groups there may be imbalances between the groups in terms of age, sex, level of disability, rate of disease progression, etc. unless the patients have been carefully matched.

Certain limitations, then, must be borne in mind when considering the conclusions reached using this trial design. As this design relies on the random nature of the group, the conclusions about a treatment can only be generalized to the group. The more random the group the greater the diversity of symptoms and, therefore, a statement can only be made about the response of the group overall and not whether a treatment is beneficial for the individual patient. Even when all participants of the group are similar for certain character-istics the conclusions can only be applied to those who match the group characteristics. The group trial is inflexible because it cannot take into account the needs of the individual on a treatment basis as would happen in a clinical setting, or make any use of odd or extreme results, as these figures would simply be averaged into the overall figures. In addition, when group data is analysed, the deterioration of some individuals will cancel the improvements made by others. Again, in effect, this only allows statements about the overall effect of a treatment on the group. The clinical trial is best suited to answer questions about group responses or when trying to determine the extent of a particular treatment effect such as the percentage of patients who are likely to respond to a specific treatment.

The single case experimental design may be more suitable for studies with MS patients, as it immediately overcomes some of the problems described above. The basis of the design is the establishment of a baseline, followed by a treatment phase, and then withdrawal of treatment back to baseline conditions (the A-B-A design). With this design one can see immediately cause and effect relationships with a particular treatment, as improvements seen when treatment commences should return to baseline levels when that treatment is withdrawn. More complex design strategies are available for studies where the A-B-A design may not be adequate, e.g. when evaluating treatments that have different therapeutic components, variations in procedures or effects that cannot be withdrawn. For a further discussion of this subject see Barlow and Hersen (1984).

This design allows greater flexibility as only small numbers are needed and the subject acts as his or her own control. When patients respond differently to a treatment, one can immediately investigate the reasons for this variability, and results can be used immediately to adjust treatment programmes. It is sometimes difficult for a single case design to be double-blind, but rigorous assessment procedures can overcome this. Conclusions can only be applied to the individual being investigated, and cannot be generalized to a larger group. However, by clearly defining individual characteristics that may be relevant to a treatment's success, and then repeating the single case study on similar individuals, one can approach generality. This design is particularly suited to answering questions about the individual. Is the patient improving? If so, by how much, and if not, what are the reasons? It is easily applied to a clinical setting and is a good technique for establishing cause and effect with the individual case. One can investigate whether changes in treatment might bring about more rapid improvement or what part other therapies may play in the improvement.

IS THE CHANGE RELEVANT TO THE PATIENT?

'. . . The treatment and management of illness is something which all societies have to provide in one way or another. But in order to make that provision as appropriate and effective as possible, it is necessary for research to go beyond what is happening in the body into the realms of behavior, beliefs and social actions . . .' (Brunel-Arms Research Unit, 1986; p.5).

In chronic conditions, for treatments to be considered successful, they must be utilized consistently and long term by the patient in addition to having been shown to be successful in a trial. The extent to which a patient complies to a treatment programme is partly determined by his/her beliefs about their responsibility for health, their views about changes brought about by a treatment, and the effects on their life style. These issues may be approached in the clinical setting, but may often leave both the clinician and the patient confused and frustrated because there is no framework for dealing with areas that are difficult to measure. But in a clinical trial to determine the effectiveness of a treatment these areas are seldom explored. Rigorous procedures must be adhered to in research to eliminate patient and observer bias and for comparability with other trials. But the very nature of the methods employed often excludes certain types of information from being used, such as patients' self-reports of the effects they have experienced from treatment. This is at variance with the clinical setting where the doctor or therapist often relies on the patient's report of any effects to adjust the treatment regimen.

Part of the problem lies in the assessment techniques themselves. The changes brought about by treatment have to be observable by others and measurable on valid and acceptable scales. Patients' own reports are not so easily quantifiable and thus many trials exclude them. Where they are included it is often as an aside to the objective assessment techniques used, and the patients' own views of changes may in fact even contradict the findings of the objective tests. These discrepancies between objective and subjective findings are often explained as patient expectation of the treatment, with interpretation going no further. The result is the loss of valuable information. Wynne (1989) has suggested that in a clinical trial involving a group of MS patients, the researchers and the patients may give different interpretation to any changes that occur when considering the efficacy of a particular treatment. Thus, the researcher looks at symptoms which can be measured, while the patient looks at daily experiences which can all be affected by treatment.

On what criteria, then, is a therapy considered to be effective? Has effectiveness been defined from physical changes that can be measured or from the patient's point of view? And is it the researcher, the clinician or the patient who makes this judgement?

A recent double-blind controlled trial investigating the efficacy of HBO in MS (Worthington *et al.*, 1987) incorporated into the trial design the collection and analysis of patient self-assessments (Monks, 1988; Wynne, 1989). This trial pursued some of the above questions by asking the patients their views in their own terms, and raised a number of issues concerning the way patients evaluate a particular therapy's effectiveness.

On the objective measurements overall the trial showed little difference between the treatment and control groups, but 23 out of 44 participants decided to continue HBO. One reason for this may be that patients define beneficial effects of a treatment in different terms. Monks (1988) found that '. . . a range of subjective measures indicated perceived benefit (although not related to HBO *per se*) without concurrent medical corroboration. That this perceived benefit was an important factor in the decision to continue with therapy seemed to indicate that it carried personal significance.' Patients will consider both the positive and negative aspects of a treatment in making a decision whether or not to continue, and may view a treatment as being useful for non-medical reasons. Monks (1988) reported a significant relationship ($P < 0.008$) between improvement in social isolation scores and continuing treatment. Other reasons for discontinuing a treatment include cost of treatment, length of travelling and involvement of other family members. The subjective data showed, however, that for the patient, beneficial effects were not always those taken into consideration during the trial. For example, improvements in appetite, the ability to do more housework, and being more clear-headed were seen as signs of HBO's effect on their condition (Wynne, 1989). Treatment was also seen as beneficial even if no direct effects were felt because it may be working as a preventative agent (Wynne, 1989). Participants also stated that involvement with HBO had caused them to realize they could do more than they thought, thus perhaps improving their mental outlook. This then could indirectly affect their MS which was seen as a valid benefit (Wynne, 1989).

Wynne (1989) also found that the patients' own evaluation of a treatment is a complex process and that research is judged in two ways. Each individual judged whether HBO had affected them personally, often over a different time frame from that imposed by a trial. This can mean looking for changes in daily symptom patterns rather than at fixed time points, correlating changes to months before the trial rather than the previous assessment. At the same time, patients realize that the effects of therapy were individual and what worked for one person may not be appropriate for another and vice versa. And thus for this reason it was not seen as contradictory if the formal results of the objective measures did not corroborate their own findings. It would appear, then, that patients evaluate a

185

treatment's effectiveness on different grounds to that of the clinical trial, and this will partly determine whether a treatment is successfully utilized.

Ultimately, however, treatment must be successful from the clinical rather than research point of view, both for the patient and for the medical practitioner or therapist. However, several points should be borne in mind.

Beneficial results of a trial are not always replicated in the clinic for several reasons. In group trials the findings are generalized to the group as a whole and may not apply to all individuals. Also the rigour of research conditions is not always met in a treatment setting, thus affecting the outcome of the treatment. Research findings need to be made more applicable to the clinical setting. When a new treatment is to be used the paper should be reviewed carefully so that the conclusions can be accurately applied to the clinical setting. If the trial conclusions are found to translate into a suitable goal of treatment in the clinic then parameters of treatment should start with those used in the trial. Patients undergoing treatment, both at the clinic and at home, must be supervised to ensure compliance as participation in research often in itself increases compliance. If the trial has concluded with a description of patients who have responded well to the experimental treatment then these selection criteria should be used when first applying the treatment in a clinical setting.

One should bear in mind, however, that the advantage of the clinical setting is its flexibility, which allows treatment to be adapted to each individual's needs. By making treatment more relevant to each individual the success rate of a particular treatment can be increased. The treatment can then be evaluated on an individual basis using the single case experimental design in the clinic, thus corroborating or refining the original results.

MS is a progressive disease and, therefore, treatment will fail from the patients' point of view if they see the goal of the treatment as a cure of the disease. If the goal is to slow progression, increase functional ability or improve symptom management then this must be clearly defined for the patient. This, then, identifies both a specific goal and a finite amount of time in which to reach that goal. The amount of benefit obtained with a particular treatment can then be measured against this goal to determine whether or not treatment has been successful.

It is also important to understand the patients' views in evaluating both response and compliance to treatment. We, as clinical practitioners, apply treatments and therapies to patients that we believe to be beneficial. We decide which treatment or therapy to give based more or less on our clinical experience and from reports in the literature. We, then, expect the patient to cooperate with the treatment, either take the tablets, change their diet, or follow a home exercise regimen. But medications have side-effects, dietary changes may conflict with life style and commitment to daily exercise requires motivation.

What this should emphasize is that decisions surrounding treatment, especially for chronic diseases, involve a complex set of issues. Treatment must be flexible and evolve as the disease progresses or the patient's life style changes. In many cases there is not only one treatment under consideration. Treatment for chronic diseases is often a mixture of therapies which must fit into an already existing life style. Ideally, treatments should fit into an overall plan of disease management which can be incorporated by each patient into their life. Therapy must involve discussion with the patient of their needs and of this overall plan to determine the appropriate approach. In the end the patient will ultimately decide which treatment and therapies are relevant to their condition. These decisions will be based on how a particular treatment affects their everyday life, their health beliefs, and how well they have understood the need for an overall plan of disease management. On the other hand, the health practitioner is responsible for this health education process, providing clear and accurate information regarding a treatment, its effects, side-effects, and consequences of not doing the treatment.

REFERENCES

Barlow, D.H. and Hersen, M. (1984) *Single Case Experimental Designs. Strategies for studying behavior change.* Pergamon Press, New York.

Brunel-Arms Research Unit (1986) *Measuring Effects. General report number 4.* Action and Research for Multiple Sclerosis (ARMS) Pubs.

Conrad, P. (1985) The meaning of medication: another look at compliance. *Social Science and Medicine,* **20**, 29–37.

McDowell, I. and Nevell, C. (1987) *Measuring Health. A guide to rating scales and questionnaires.* Oxford University Press, Oxford.

McEwen, J. (1983) The Nottingham Health Profile: A measure of perceived health, in *Measuring the social benefits of medicine* (ed. G. Teeling Smith). Office of Health Economics.

Monks, J. (1988) Interpretation of subjective measures in a clinical trial of hyperbaric oxygen therapy for multiple sclerosis. *Journal of Psychosomatic Research,* **32**, 365–72.

Poser, C.M., Paty, D.W., Scheinberg, L. *et al.* (1984) New diagnostic criteria for multiple sclerosis, in *The Diagnosis of Multiple Sclerosis* (ed. C.M. Poser). Thieme-Stratton Inc., New York, pp. 225–9.

Waksman, B.H. (1983) Rationales of current therapies of multiple sclerosis. *Archives of Neurology,* **40**, 671–2.

Weiner, L. and Ellison, G.W. (1983) A working protocol to be used as a guideline for trials in multiple sclerosis. *Archives of Neurology,* **40**, 704–10.

Worthington, J.A., De Souza, L.H., Forti, A. *et al.* (1987) A double-blind controlled cross-over trial investigating the efficacy of hyperbaric oxygen in patients with multiple sclerosis, in *Multiple Sclerosis: Immunological, Diagnostic and Therapeutic Aspects* (eds F. Clifford Rose and R. Jones). John Libbey and Company Ltd., London, pp. 229–40.

Wynne, A. (1989) Is it any good? The evaluation of therapy by participants in a clinical trial. *Social Science and Medicine,* **29**(11), 1289–97.

Index